P. A. Foster   J. A. Roelofse

Databook of Anaesthesia and Critical Care Medicine

Fourth, Revised and Enlarged Edition

Springer-Verlag
Berlin Heidelberg New York
London Paris Tokyo

Prof. Dr. Patrick Anthony Foster Dr. James A. Roelofse
University of Stellenbosch, Faculty of Medicine,
Department of Anaesthesia, P.O. Box 63,
ZA-7505 Tygerberg, South Africa

The three previous editions were published in 1978, 1980, and 1982 by
Medishield Corporation Limited, London.

ISBN 3-540-17794-9 Springer-Verlag Berlin Heidelberg New York
ISBN 0-387-17794-9 Springer-Verlag New York Berlin Heidelberg

Library of Congress Cataloging in Publication Data. Main entry under title:
Foster, P.A. (Patrick Anthony), Databook of anaesthesia and critical care medicine. Bibliography:
p. 1. Anesthesiology. 2. Critical care medicine. I. Roelofse, J.A. (James A.), 1942- . II. Title.
[DNLM: 1. Anesthesiology-handbooks. 2. Critical Care-handbooks. WO 231 F756d] RD82.F67
1987 617'.96 87-9653

© Springer-Verlag Berlin Heidelberg 1987
   Printed in Germany

Typesetting, printing, and bookbinding: Appl, Wemding

2119/3140-543210

Preface to the Fourth Edition

This book is intended to bring together data and clinical guidelines for those involved in the practice of anaesthesia, whether they be specialists or not. It is designed to be a true handbook that will accompany its owner into the operating theatre, where it will serve as a practical reference guide, not as a textbook.

We welcome comment, criticism, and suggestions for improvement of the contents; correspondence may be addressed to the authors at P.O. Box 63, Tygerberg 7505, Republic of South Africa.

We wish to acknowledge help received from our colleagues over the years of publication: Dr. T.J.V. Voss, Prof. G.G. Harrison, Dr. C.M. Lewis, Dr. W.B. Murray, Prof. A.R. Coetzee, and Dr. W.L. van der Merwe.

Acknowledgement is also made to "Anaesthesia Guidelines", long since out of print, on which the first edition of this handbook was based in 1978.

Tygerberg, South Africa, May 1987   *P.A. Foster*
                                                J.A. Roelofse

Contents

Chapter 3

Chapter 4

Chapter 1

I. Pre-anaesthetic Assessment and Preparation

A. Anaesthetic Risk Assessment

1. New York Heart Association Functional Classification

Class 1   No limitation of activity
Class 2   Some limitation of heavy exertion, but can walk three blocks without shortness of breath, or climb a flight of stairs (3 m)
Class 3   Some limitation of ordinary activity, with difficulty in walking three blocks or climbing a flight of stairs
Class 4   Shortness of breath at rest

2. ASA Classification of Physical Status

Class I   Normal healthy patient
Class II   A patient with mild systemic disease
Class III A patient with systemic disease severe enough to limit activity but not incapacitating
Class IV A patient with severe incapacitating systemic disease that is a constant threat to life
Class V   Moribund patient not expected to survive 24 h with our without surgery
E   Emergency operation – the symbol "E" is appended to the appropriate classification

The ASA classification has limitations for predicting anaesthetic and surgical risk, owing to the omission of important factors such as extremes of age, duration of surgery, immediate preoperative investigations and treatments, and the competence of the surgeon. The following classification, adapted from Prof. Lutz (Mannheim), includes most important risk factors.

Score the appropriate points in each section and total:

0	1	2	3	4
Planned operation				
Outpatient		Semi-emer-gency		Emergency
Inpatient				
Operation site				
		Thoracic	Aorta	
		Abdominal		
Length of operation				
< 120 min	120–180 min	> 180 min		
Age				
1–39 years	40–59 years	> 59 years		
General status				
Good	Chronic wasting disease	Confined to bed		Acute life-threatening condition Shock Resp. failure
CNS				
Fully conscious				unconscious
Cardiac status				
Normal	Low exercise tolerance	Cardiomegaly	Pulmonary congestion	
No coronary disease	Acrocyanosis	Dependent oedema	Infarct < 6 mo, 2 or more pre-vious infarcts	
	Digitalis	Raised JVP		
	Cardiac abnormality	Angina		
		Endocardial in-jury on ECG		
		Infarct 6–12 mo		
Cardiac rhythm				
Normal	Not sinus rhythm	Tachycardia > 120		
	AV block 1st or 2nd degree	Supraventri-cular extra-systoles		
	Total RBB block	Ventricular extrasystoles		
		LBB block		

0	1	2	3	4
Circulation				
No significant problem	Hypertension > 145/95	Arteriosclerosis Dehydration – diuretics, starvation, bowel washout		
Respiration				
Normal	Acute bronchitis Chronic bronchitis Emphysema	Bronchospasm	Pneumonia Dyspnoea of resp. origin	
Metabolism				
Normal	Overweight > 30%	Diabetes mellitus		
Serum potassium				
Normal		Serum K + > 5 mmol/l < 3 mmol/l		
Haemoglobin				
> 12.5 g%		< 12.5 g%		
Liver function				
Normal		Raised transaminase Raised gamma GT Lowered Quick's test Cirrhosis Low cholinesterase		
Renal function				
Normal		Raised urea/BUN		

Risk groups	0–6 Low risk 7–10 medium risk > 10 High risk

B. Cardiac Risk Index (according to Goldman et al. [8]

Risk is assessed by totaling the points scored under the following headings:

1. History
   - Age > 70 years — 5
   - Myocardial infarct within past 6 months — 10 (15)

2. Physical examination
   - Valvular aortic stenosis — 3
   - Third heart sound or raised JVP — 11 (14)

3. ECG
   - Recent ECG shows rhythm other than sinus, or atrial extrasystoles — 7
   - > 5 ventricular extrasystoles per min at any time preoperatively — 7 (14)

4. Biochemistry
   - PaO_2 < 60 mmHg (8 kPa)
   - $PaCO_2$ > 50 mmHg (6.5 kPa)
   - Blood urea > 6.5 mmol/l — for any
   - Serum potassium < 3.0 mmol/l — 3
   - Plasma HCO_3 < 20 mmol/l
   - Serum creatinine > 3.0 mg/dl — (18)

5. Proposed surgery
   - Intraperitoneal, intrathoracic or aortic — 3
   - Emergency surgery — 4
   - Duration of surgery beyond 2 h — 3 (10)

Risk assessment using the above factors:

Score	Evaluation	Prediction of serious complication (%)	Predicted mortality (%)
5	Normal	0.7	0.2
6–13	Critical	5.0	2.0
13–25	Needs specific consultation for cardiac problems	11.0	2.0
> 25	Elective surgery not justified without specific reason	22.0	56

C. Respiratory Risk Assessment

1. Poor Prognostic Signs

General   Rapid shallow breathing
Alae nasi movement
Cyanosis
Cough and sputum before abdominal or thoracic surgery
Pyrexia
Anaemia

PaO_2 < 9 kPa (70 mm Hg) breathing air

$PaCO_2$ > 6.5 kPa (50 mmH g)

MBC $< 50\%$ of predicted or 70 l/min will have 50% mortality

FEV_1 < 2 litres   – high risk

         < 1 litre   – exclude from general anaesthetic

FVC < 2 litres   – postoperative problem

         < 1.5 litre   – ineffective cough

         < 1 litre   – will need postoperative assistance

2. Normal Respiratory Function Values for the Average Young Adult

Total lung compliance	100 ml/cm H_2O or $0.05 \times FRC$ litres per cm H_2O
Work of breathing	0.5 kg/m/min or 0.5–1.0 ml O_2 per litre breathed
V_d/V_t (dead space)	$< 30\%$
MBC	120 l/min or $35 \times FEV_1$
FEV_1	83% or better
Alveolar ventilation	2.0–2.5 l/min/m²
Minute volume	5–8 l/min (adult)
Mean mechanical resistance	0.6–2.4 cm H_2O/l/s
Pulmonary diffusing capacity (carbon monoxide)	17–25 ml/min/mm Hg²
Peak expiratory flow rate	$4–5 \times MBC$
Dead space calculations	

– Anatomical dead space $= TV \left(\dfrac{\text{end expired } pCO_2 - \text{mixed expired } pCO_2}{\text{end expired } pCO_2 - \text{inspired } pCO_2} \right)$

– Physiological dead space $= Vt \left(\dfrac{PaCO_2 - PeCO_2}{PaCO_2} \right)$

D. Hepatic Reserve and Anaesthetic Risk

1. Child's System [30]

	Class A	Class B	Class C
Serum bilirubin (μmol/l)	40	40–50	50
Serum albumin (g/l)	35	30–35	30
Ascites	None	Easy control	Poor control
Neurological disorder	None	Minimal	Advanced coma
Nutrition	Excellent	Good	Poor with wasting
Risk of operation	Good	Moderate	Poor

2. Pugh's System

	Points scored for increasing abnormalities		
	1	2	3
Serum bilirubin (μmol/l)	25	25–40	40
Serum albumin (g/l)	35	28–35	28
Prothrombin time increase over control in seconds	1–4	4–6	6
Encephalopathy (grade)	None	1 & 2	3 & 4
Risk of operation	Good	Moderate	Poor

5– 6 points: good operative risk (equivalent to Child's class A)
7– 9 points: moderate operative risk (equivalent to Child's class B)
10–15 points: poor operative risk (equivalent to Child's class C)

E. Pre-anaesthetic Check List

Before first case of day

1. Check out machine

  a) pipeline connections correct, use oxygen analyser
  b) gas supply (O_2, N_2O reserve tanks)
  c) vaporizers filled with correct drug
  d) test breathing circuits for leaks: Obstruct patient connexion, pressurize the circuit to 30 cm H_2O, observe manometer for leak. Any leakage rate can be measured by adjusting a flowmeter to maintain a constant pressure. This leakage should be less than 100 ml/min.
  e) breathe through system – check valve movement and seating
  f) ventilator functioning
  g) suction operative

    h) check scavenging system
    i) absorber operative
    j) humidifier temperature correct
2. *Check and calibrate monitors*
    a) sphygmomanometer/oscillotonometer
    b) peripheral pulse monitor
    c) electrocardiogram
    d) all pressure transducers at zero
    e) thermometers
    f) other transducers
3. *Check emergency drug supply*
    a) lignocaine
    b) sodium bicarbonate
    c) cardiotonics (isoprenaline, adrenaline, dopamine)
    d) propranolol
    e) atropinc
    f) vasoconstrictors
    g) calcium chloride
    h) calcium channel blocker

Before each case of day

1. *Recheck equipment*
    a) recheck machine for leaks
    b) flowmeters and vaporizers off
    c) prepare intravenous infusion devices
    d) check laryngoscope
    e) prepare minimum drugs and label – i.v. induction agent, relaxant, atropine, i.v. opiate, vasopressor
    f) prepare anaesthetic chart
2. *Patient arrives; check*
    a) identification, consent
    b) nothing per mouth for more than 6 h
    c) permits for surgery and anaesthesia
    d) premedications and effect
    e) special orders (steroids, diabetics, etc.)
    f) any lab work not available previous day
    g) status of ordered blood
    h) dentures
    i) check intravenous lines and contents
    j) roentgenograms available
    k) record patient data

3. *Attach*
   a) sphygmomanometer
   b) precordial stethoscope
   c) i.v. line and i.a. line where indicated
   d) electrocardiogram (except for special cases) and other required monitors
4. *Check all monitors – record initial values*
5. *Position patient for induction*
   a) prevent nerve injury
   b) use comfortable restraints as indicated
   c) prevent heat loss
   d) look for possible pressure points
   e) eye protection

F. Detailed Check of Anaesthetic Machine

1. *Check pipeline:*
   a) Disconnect all lines
   b) Connect oxygen, check flowmeter
   c) Check outflow gas with O_2 analyser (or inhale)
   d) Connect N_2O, check flowmeter
   e) Disconnect oxygen, check O_2 failure device if fitted
2. *Check cylinder:*
   a) Open all fresh cylinders to clear outlet before connecting
   b) Check correct match of cylinder to connector
   c) Always open flowmeter before opening cylinder
   d) Check all cylinder pressures: gauge pressure indicates contents only for O_2 or AIR, but not for N_2O, CO_2, C_3H_6. Label "FULL" and "IN USE" clinders – open "IN USE" only
3. *Check flowmeters:*
   a) All bobbins operate smoothly over full range, return to zero
   b) Check control knobs for sensitivity, spindle alignment, other damage
   c) Close all gases
4. *Check vaporizers:*
   a) Check fluid level and colour; refill if necessary
   b) Check operation of vaporizer control, and switch off
   c) Open one flowmeter, occlude machine outlet, check for vaporizer leaks

Method: Obstruct machine outlet; briefly pressurize circuit to 30 cm H$_2$O and switch off gas; pressure should stay constant

    d) Check operation of minimum oxygen percentage mixer if fitted

5. *Check breathing circuit:*

    a) General test

       Method: Obstruct patient connexion, pressurize the circuit to 30 cm H$_2$O, observe manometer for leak. Any leakage rate can be measured by adjusting a flowmeter to maintain a constant pressure. This leakage should be less than 100 ml/min

    b) Specific tests

       Bain (Mapleson D mod.) – check expiratory valve

       Occlude internal pipe outflow, check for leaks

       Magill (Mapleson A) – check expiratory valve

       Ayre's T-piece (Mapleson E) – expiratory limb open

       Circle absorber – prime with oxygen, check for leaks and expiratory valve

       Check absorber on/off control

       Bag on patient connexion – check that unidirectional valves work correctly

       Check colour-change sequence of soda lime

       Check soda lime colour, particle size

       Periodically check for soda lime dust accumulation

6. *All circuits:*

    Occlude outlet, distend rebreathing bag, check for slow leaks

    Check bag for damage

    If circuit pressure gauge fitted, check opening pressure of expiratory valve

7. *Use oxygen analyser to check outflowing mixture before use –*
    are flowmeters accurate?

8. *Check flowrate of emergency oxygen*
    Fill 2-litre bag in ± 5 s $= 24$ l/min

9. *Check ventilator:*

    Check and set volume

    Check inspiratory time, expiratory time, minute rate

    Connect to breathing circuit with reservoir bag as "patient lung", check function

    Check circuit pressure gauge for zero set, damage

    Check ventilator dump port open (scavenging port included)

    Know your ventilator

    Check how to switch to hand control

10. *Double-check any newly serviced equipment before use on any patient*

G. Requirements for Paediatric Anaesthesia

Requirements

1. Establish correct weight, blood volume, appropriate doses of parenteral drugs
2. Correct breathing circuits, endotracheal tubes and connectors, laryngoscope
3. Accurate low-flow flowmeters and vaporizers
4. Establish i.v. line, accurate small-volume measuring i.v. sets
5. Correct size sphygmomanometer cuff – Doppler flow detector
6. Protection against heat loss:
   - sterile cotton wool insulation
   - warm-water blanket
   - heated humidifier in circuit
   - correct ambient temperature $> 22\,°C$, ideal $> 26\,°C$
   - in-line i.v. fluid warmer
7. Oesophageal thermometer
8. Oesophageal precordial stethoscope
9. Equipment for measuring blood loss
10. i.v. infusion-rate controller
11. Monitors:
    - peripheral pulse
    - ECG
    - infant capnograph
    - peripheral nerve stimulator
12. Suction equipment with small catheters, vacuum control
13. Good assistance
14. Prearrange for recovery area reception

Special Problems in Paediatrics

1. Handling of drugs may vary due to:
   - unsophisticated hepatic enzymes
   - large extracellular fluid volume
2. Response to muscle relaxants:
   - sensitive to non-depolarizers
   - resistant to depolarizers
3. Sensitive to barbiturates, opiates, benzodiazepines
4. Rate of uptake of inhalation anaesthetics is more rapid than in adult
5. Local anaesthetics more prone to produce cardiovascular depression
6. Poor postoperative body temperature control, use incubator, set at $32\,°C$, humidity 65%

7. Do not exceed FIO_2 0.4 – danger of retrolental fibroplasia
8. Observe sterile practice – unsophisticated immune system
9. Poor cough reflex, narrow airways easily obstructed by secretions, mucous membrane swelling

H. Ventilator Settings in Paediatric Circuits

Prediction of child's minute volume
a. Minute Volume (V_e) = Tidal volume (V_t) × Frequency/min (f)
b. Tidal Volume (V_t) = Body mass (kg) × 8
c. Frequency/min (f) varies with mass decreasing with age

Body Mass kg	Tidal volume (kg × 8)	Frequency/min f	Minute volume V_e
2	16 ml	30	480 ml
3	24 ml	25	600 ml
10	80 ml	21	1700 ml
20	160 ml	19	3000 ml
30	240 ml	17	4000 ml
40	320 ml	15	4800 ml
50	400 ml	13	5200 ml
60	480 ml	11	5300 ml
70	560 ml	10	5600 ml

Infants and Children to the age of 5 (alternative system) [21]
d. Tidal volume 4.3 ml/kg ($V_t = 4.11 \times kg + 1.58$ [r = 0.94])
    Minute volume $V_e = 120 \times kg + 560$ [r = 0.81]
e. Dynamic compliance 10 ml/Pa/kg

I. Ventilator Settings in Adult Circuits

Fresh gas flow required to provide normal $PaCO_2$ with non-rebreathing breathing circuits

Type of system	Spontaneous breathing	IPPV = $\dot{V}$	IPPV > V*
Magill	V × 1	V × 2 +	N.A.
Potter's valve and mask	V × 2	N.A.	N.A.
T-piece, e.g. Ayre, Bain, Rees	V × 2.5	V × 2	V × 1
Cape Town	V × 3	N.A.	N.A.

* Hyperventilation while maintaining normal $PaCO_2$
  Oxygen content of mixture never below 30%

J. Guidelines for Endotracheal Tube Sizes (mm ID)

Age (years)	Prem.	0	3 mos	1	2	3	4.5	6	9	12
Size	2.5	3	3.5	4	4.5	5	5.5	6	7	7.5
Orotracheal length	8.5	9.5	10.5	12	13	13.5	14	15	16	18
Nasotracheal length		11.5	12.5	14	15	15.5	16	17	19	21

Age (years)	15	Adult ♀	Adult ♂
Size	7.5– 8.0	7.5– 8.5	8–10
Orotracheal length	18 –23	23 –26	23–26
Nasotracheal length	24 –30	30 –36	30–36

Notes:

A. The cricoid cartilage is narrower than the vocal cords that you can see.

B. The correct size is always a loose fitting through the cricoid cartilage.

C. Never use a cuffed endotracheal tube in children under 10 years of age.

D. In children under 3, both main bronchi come off the trachea at an equal angle.

E. In neonates, the laryngeal opening is anterior and high, opposite C2–4. The angle between epiglottis and tongue is 45°.
   Glottic opening is funnel shaped.

General guideline above 3 years
   Oral endotracheal tube   d × 1.5
   Nasal endotracheal Tube   d × 2.0

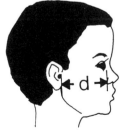

Notes:

1. Always auscultate both lungs after placement of the tube.

2. Flexion and extension of the head and insertion of mouth gags changes the level of the endotracheal tube in the trachea.

3. Mark the endotracheal tube 2.2 cm from its tip. Fix the tube when this mark is at the vocal cords.

K. Catheter Sizes

Endotracheal tube sizes refer to the internal diameter. Wall thickness varies with tube diameter and material used between 1.0 and 2.2 mm. A nominal average external diameter is given. All measurements are in mm.

Endotracheal tube internal diameter	Typical external diameter	French gauge
11.0	15.3	46
10.5	14.7	44
10.0	14.0	42
9.5	13.3	40
9.0	12.7	38
8.5	12.0	36
8.0	11.3	34
7.5	10.7	32
7.0	10.0	30
6.5	9.3	28
6.0	8.7	26
5.5	8.0	24
5.0	7.3	22
4.5	6.7	20
4.0	6.0	18
3.5	5.3	16
3.0	4.7	14
2.5	4.0	12
2.0	3.3	10
1.5	2.7	8
	2.3	7
	2.0	6
	1.7	5
	1.3	4
	1.0	3
	0.7	2
	0.3	1

L. Hypodermic Needle Gauges

British wire gauge	Diameter (mm)
28	0.35
27	0.40
26	0.45
25	0.50
24	0.55
23	0.60
22	0.70
21	0.80
20	0.90
19	1.10
18	1.25
17	1.45
16	1.65
15	1.80
14	2.10

M. Particle Sizes

Filters are used in breathing circuits and infusion lines during anaesthesia. The pore size is defined by the manufacturer, and will generally be uniform only in screen filters but not random fibre filters. The diameter of various particles that may need filtration is given in micrometer (μm).

Viruses	0.003–0.06
Tobacco smoke	0.01–1.0
Carbon black	0.01–0.3
Pleuropneumonia-like organisms	0.12–0.25
Pseudomonas diminuta	0.3
Serratia marcescens	0.5
Bacteria	0.3–30
Lung-damaging dust	0.5–5
Jeweller's rouge	1–10
Ultrasonically generated fogs	2–80
Peripheral capillaries	4
Yeasts	6
Red blood cells	7
Lung capillaries	8
Lung arterioles	35–50

Pollens	10–100
Smallest visible particle	40
Human hair	±75
Mist	80–200
Standard blood filter	170–230

Red blood corpuscles deform in traversing peripheral capillaries unless they are hypoxic, in which case the cell wall becomes stiff.

N. Mortality and Morbidity

A classification of mortality and morbidity related to surgery and anaesthesia [18]

Deaths related to surgery
1. Attributable to anaesthesia
2. Not attributable to anaesthesia
   a) Surgical
   b) Other
      – disease
      – not assessable

Deaths to anaesthesia attributable
1. Failure of organization
2. Failure of equipment
3. Drug effect (excluding overdose)
4. Human error – anaesthetist failure
   a) Lack of knowledge
   b) Lack of care
   c) Failure to apply knowledge
   d) Lack of experience
   e) Other
      – fatigue
      – impairment – mental illness
                    – physical illness
                    – drug-induced

Morbidity related to surgery

Major:	Causes permanent disability or disfigurement
Intermediate:	Causes serious distress and/or prolongation of hospital stay, but no permanent sequelae
Minor:	Causes moderate distress without prolongation of hospital stay or permanent sequelae

O. Postoperative Recovery Score

Sign	Criterion	Score
Consciousness	Awake, communicating	2
	Responds to stimuli	1
	Not responding	0
Airway	Talking, coughing on request, crying	2
	Maintains own airway	1
	Airway needs maintenance	0
Movement	Purposeful movement	2
	Non-purposeful movement	1
	Not moving	0
Local analgesia	Full sensory recovery	2
	Sensory block present	1
	Sensory and motor block	0
Circulation	Systolic BP within ±20% of pre-op	2
	Systolic BP ±20%–50% of pre-op	1
	Systolic BP >50% deviation from pre-op	0
Skin colour	Warm and pink	2
	Pale, dusky, blotchy	1
	Cyanotic	0

Criteria for discharge after day case surgery:
- Patient can stand for 1 min with eyes closed and without hypotension >20 mm Hg systolic
- More than 1 h has passed after surgery under GA
- Patient has taken liquids with sugar by mouth
- Half-life of i.v. drugs influences fitness for discharge

Following discharge after day case surgery, subject should not:
- Walk in street alone or on high walkways
- Use alcohol or other sedatives unless supervised
- Work with power tools
- Drive an automobile
- Make important decisions
- Indulge in strenuous exercise

II. Anaesthetic Physical Constants

A. Physical Properties of Inhalational Agents

Agent	Formula	Structure
(A) Methoxyflurane	$C_3H_4OCl_2F_2$	$\begin{array}{ccc} Cl & F & H \\ \mid & \mid & \mid \\ H-C-C-O-C-H \\ \mid & \mid & \mid \\ Cl & F & H \end{array}$
(B) Trichlorethylene	C_2HCl_3	$\begin{array}{cc} H & Cl \\ \mid & \mid \\ C=C \\ \mid & \mid \\ Cl & Cl \end{array}$
(C) Chloroform	$CHCl_3$	$\begin{array}{c} Cl \\ \mid \\ H-C-Cl \\ \mid \\ Cl \end{array}$
(D) Halothane	$C_2HClBrF_3$	$\begin{array}{cc} Br & F \\ \mid & \mid \\ H-C-C-F \\ \mid & \mid \\ Cl & F \end{array}$
(E) Enflurane	$C_3H_2OClF_5$	$\begin{array}{ccc} F & F & F \\ \mid & \mid & \mid \\ H-C-C-O-C-H \\ \mid & \mid & \mid \\ Cl & F & F \end{array}$
(F) Isoflurane	$C_3H_2OClF_5$	$\begin{array}{ccc} F & Cl & F \\ \mid & \mid & \mid \\ F-C-C-O-C-H \\ \mid & \mid & \mid \\ F & H & F \end{array}$

	Agent	Formula	Structure
Ⓖ	Diethylether	$C_4H_{10}O$	H H H H | | | | H—C—C—O—C—C—H | | | | H H H H
Ⓗ	Fluroxene	$C_4H_5OF_3$	F H H H | | | | F—C—C—O—C=C—H | | F H
Ⓘ	Ethylchloride	C_2H_5Cl	H H | | H—C—C—Cl | | H H
Ⓙ	Divinylether	C_4H_6O	H H H H | | | | C=C—O—C= C | | H H
Ⓚ	Xenon	Xe	
Ⓛ	Cyclopropane	C_3H_6	CH_2 / \\ CH_2 — CH_2
Ⓜ	Ethylene	C_2H_4	H H | | C=C | | H H
Ⓝ	Nitrous oxide	N_2O	$N \equiv N = O$

	mol. wt.	sg	LH cal/mole	bp	kPa VP 20°C
Ⓐ	165	1.42	9.43	104.7	3
Ⓑ	131.4	1.46	8.004	86.8	7.7
Ⓒ	119	1.47	8.617	61.2	20
Ⓓ	197.4	1.86	6.77	50	32.3
Ⓔ	184.5	1.52	6.74	56.5	24
Ⓕ	184.5	1.49	7.39	48.5	33.2
Ⓖ	74.1	0.72	6.4	34.6	58.8
Ⓗ	126.0	1.13	6.524	43.2	38
Ⓘ	64.52	0.92		12.4	133.4
Ⓙ	70.10	0.77	6.3	28.3	77
Ⓚ	131	4.53 (air)	3.11	−108	Gas above crit. temp.
Ⓛ	42.0	1.45 (air)	4.8	−33	746
Ⓜ	28	0.9 (air)	3.5	−103.7	5.81
Ⓝ	44	1.5 (air)	3.958	−88.5	5305

	25°C MAC mg/ml gas	37°C MAC	Water solubility	Olive oil	Blood	Critical Temperature °C	Critical Pressure mPa
Ⓐ	6.75	0.16	3.5	930	13		
Ⓑ	5.38	0.23	1.51	720	9.15	271	5.0
Ⓒ	4.89	0.64	3.9	265	8.4	263	5.47
Ⓓ	8.05	0.77	0.86	224	2.3	296	3.95
Ⓔ	7.56	1.68	0.82	98.5	1.91		
Ⓕ	7.56	1.2	0.61	97.8	1.43		
Ⓖ	3.03	1.94	13	50.2	12.1	194	36
Ⓗ	5.15	3.4	0.84	56.8	1.37		
Ⓘ	1.1	3.82	1.2		3.0	187	5.27
Ⓙ	2.86	4.0	1.45	58	2.2	190	4.75
Ⓚ	5.29	71	0.097	1.93	0.17	176	5.9
Ⓛ	1.72	9.3	0.22	11.2	0.45–0.6	124.4	5.5
Ⓜ	1.16	67	0.08	1.28	0.14	9.6	5.16
Ⓝ	1.79	102	0.44	1.40	0.478	36.5	7.25

VP = Vapour pressure in kPa at 20 °C; *LH* = Latent heat of evaporation at 20 °C in Cal/mole ($\overline{v}g^{-1}$). Blood solubility is the same as blood/gas solubility coefficients; *MAC* = Minimum alveolar concentration in oxygen V/V% of 1 atmosphere (101.3 kPa) and body temperature of 37 °C.

Xenon at room temperature (20 °C) is above its critical temperature of 16.7 °C, and is thus regarded as a gas, unlike ethylene, cyclopropane, and nitrous oxide.

To derive the number of grams of vapour per litre, or mg/ml, of an anaesthetic, use Avogadro's hypothesis:

$$\frac{\text{g mol wt}}{\text{g mol vol}} = \frac{\text{col 3}}{22.4} \text{ at } 0\,°\text{C}$$

At 20 °C the factor is $\quad \text{X} \dfrac{273}{293}$

and at 37 °C $\quad \text{X} \dfrac{273}{310}$

Trooton's rule: The molar latent heat of vaporization of a liquid at its boiling point, divided by the point in degrees Kelvin (°C + 273) is a constant = ± 22.

B. Vapour Pressure Graphs

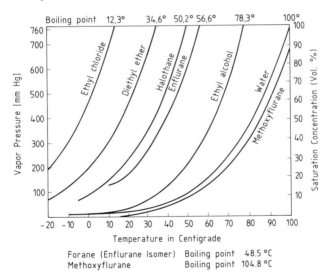

Forane (Enflurane Isomer) Boiling point 48.5 °C
Methoxyflurane Boiling point 104.8 °C

C. Volatile Anaesthetic Concentrations (Copper Kettle)

$$\% \text{ anaes } = 100 \ \frac{\dot{V}A}{\dot{V}_T} \tag{1}$$

$$= 100 \ \frac{(Pv)\dot{V}O_2 \ vap}{\dot{V}_T \ (Pb-Pv)} \tag{2}$$

$$= \frac{100\,(\dot{V}O_2 vap)\,Pv}{(\dot{V}O_2 vap)(Pb)} + (\dot{V} \ dil) \ (Pb-Pv) \tag{3}$$

where:

$\dot{V}A$ = anaesthetic vapour output (ml/min)

$\dot{V}_T$ = total vaporizing gas low (ml/min)

$\dot{V}O_2 \ vap$ = O_2 passing through vaporizer (ml/min)

$\dot{V} \ dil$ = flow of diluent gases (ml/min)

Pv = vapour pressure of volatile anaesthetic

Either formula (1), (2) or (3) may be used, depending on the information available. If $\dot{V}A$ and $\dot{V}_T$ are known, or can be approximated, then formula (1) may be used. If $\dot{V}A$ is unknown, but $\dot{V}_T$ is known, then formula (2) may be used. Formula (3) should be used when neither $\dot{V}A$ nor $\dot{V}_T$ can be approximated. For rough estimates of volatile anaesthetic concentrations, see table of anaesthetic values.

D. Vaporizer Splitting Ratios [14]

Most modern vaporizers divide the total gas flow into two components:

1. A (major) proportion that bypasses the vaporizer (B)
2. A proportion (A) that enters the vaporizing chamber to become fully saturated with a volume of vapour (C). This then rejoins and is diluted by the bypass stream.

   The fraction B/A is the *splitting ratio*. At a ratio of infinity no vapour is delivered, and maximum vapour concentration is produced at a ratio of zero when the total gas flow passes through the vaporizing chamber.

   The volume of gas leaving the vaporizer is greater than the inflow by the volume of vapour added (C).

   As the liquid temperature falls during evaporation, temperature compensation increases the flow of (B) through the vaporizing chamber to maintain a constant output.

Percentage scales on vaporizers apply only at "normal" atmospheric pressure. The saturated vapour pressure of a liquid is unaffected by changes in atmospheric pressure. If the ambient pressure falls the percentage of vapour evolved rises, but its partial pressure, on which anaesthetic effect depends, will be unchanged if the splitting ratio is constant. Theoretically, the vaporizers of more volatile liquid anaesthetics can deliver higher partial pressures at high altitudes.

Vaporization of Liquid Anaesthetics

1. Gram molecular weight produces approximately 24 litres at room temperature.

2. Vapour volume per 100 g at $20\,°C = 24 \times \dfrac{100}{\text{g mol wt}}$

3. Vapour volume per 100 ml at $20\,°C = 24 \times \dfrac{100}{\text{g mol wt}} \times \dfrac{1}{\text{sg}}$

	g mol. wt.	sg	Vapour volume	
			per 100 ml	per 100 g
Halothane	197	1.86	6.54 l	12.18 l
Enflurane	185	1.50 ⎫	19.50 l	12.90 l
Isoflurane	185	1.50 ⎭		

Liquid anaesthetic consumption ml/h at 1% vaporizer setting

Drug	Flow – l/min				
	1	2	4	5	8
1% Halothane	9	18	36	45	72
1% Enflurane	3	6	12	15	24
1% Isoflurane	3	6	12	15	24

Liquid anaesthetic consumption ml/h at 1 MAC vaporizer setting

Drug	Flow – l/min				
	1	2	4	5	8
Halothane (0.7)	6.3	12.6	25.2	31.5	50.4
Enflurane (1.68)	5	10	20	25	40
Isoflurane (1.15)	3.45	6.9	13.8	17.25	27.6

E. The Gas Laws

The standard gas laws apply to perfect gases which may be roughly equated with gaseous substances at temperatures well above their critical temperatures, or as gases in which the volume occupied by the gas molecules is small relative to the space the gas occupies. This implies negligible intermolecular forces and excludes very high pressures.

Boyle's Law: Relates pressure and volume at constant temperature. For a given mass of gas, the volume varies inversely with the pressure at constant temperature. This relationship can be mathematically expressed as a rectangular hyperbola.

Charles' Law: Relates temperature and volume at constant pressure. For a given mass of gas, the volume varies directly with the absolute temperature, at constant pressure ($0\,°C = 273°$ K). Near absolute zero this relationship does not apply, as all gases liquefy. Mathematically, this is a linear relationship.

Gay-Lussac's Law: Relates temperature and pressure at constant volume. For a given mass of gas, the pressure increases by the same percentage of its pressure at $0\,°C$ for each $1\,°C$ rise, provided the volume remains constant.

Dalton's Law of Partial Pressures: The pressure exerted by a mixture of gases, or of vapours mixed with gases, within a defined closed space is equal to the sum of the individual pressures that each constituent would exert if it alone filled the space.

Note: The compressibility of vapours and gases below or near their critical temperature does not follow Boyle's law.

Vapours: A vapour is the gaseous state of a liquid. Whether a given substance is a vapour or a gas will thus depend upon temperature. Vapours do not follow the gas laws. In a closed container, vapour pressure is only proportional to the temperature of the liquid from which it is evolved, if such a liquid reservoir is present. When the vapour pressure equals the ambient gas pressure, boiling occurs.

One gram molecular weight of a liquid when vaporized occupies 22.4 litres at 101.3 kPa and $0\,°C$, or 24 litres at 101.3 kPa and $20\,°C$.

The Ideal Gas Equation: Relates temperature, pressure and volume in a perfect gas. Based on the above three laws:

$P_1 V_1/T_1 = P_2 V_2/T_2 = $ Constant, or

$PV = nRT$ where:

P = pressure in atmospheres; V = volume (litres)
T = absolute temperature; R = the gas constant: 0.082
n = number of moles in the mass of gas under consideration

Note: Value of the gas constant depends on units of other parameters:

for N/m^2, m^3/g mol, $K°$ R = 8.314
for ATM, cm^3/g mol, $K°$ R = 82.05

Henry's Law: The mass of gas that dissolves in a given volume of solvent at a specified constant pressure is proportional to the partial pressure of the gas in contact and in equilibrium with the solvent.

Graham's Law: The rate at which different gases diffuse is inversely proportional to the square root of their molecular masses, provided all other factors are constant.

Fick's Law: The diffusion flux density is proportional to the concentration gradient. The usual unit is cm^2/s or cm^2/min.

Fick's Principle: The size of a stream can be derived from a knowledge of the amount of a substance that enters or leaves the stream at a given point, and of the resulting concentration difference in the stream.

Raoult's Law: In a solution of two liquids, the vapour pressure of each constituent is proportional to its molar concentration in unit volume of the solution. (This law applies to azeotropic mixtures which vaporize in the same ratios as their concentrations. Common azeotropes are 33% ether in 66% halothane and water in 96% ethyl alcohol).

F. Gas Cylinder Pressures and Constants

1. Physical Constants for Gases

Gas	Boiling point at atmospheric pressure	Critical temperature	Critical pressure
Nitrogen	$-195.8\,°C$	$-147.1\,°C$	3.39 mPa
Oxygen	$-183\,°C$	$-118.4\,°C$	5.08 mPa
Xenon	$-108\,°C$	$16.7\,°C$	5.88 mPa
Nitrous oxide	$-89.5\,°C$	$36.5\,°C$	7.25 mPa
Carbon dioxide sublimation pt	$-78.5\,°C$	$31\,°C$	7.38 mPa
Cyclopropane	$-32.86\,°C$	$124.4\,°C$	5.49 mPa

Standard oxygen cylinder pressure . . . . 13 600 kPa

Standard nitrous oxide cylinder pressure . . . . 5137 kPa at 21 °C (pressure varies with temperature)

1 kg of liquid $O_2 = 755$ l of gas at 21 °C

1 kg of nitrous oxide $= 540$ l of gas at 21 °C

2. Gas Cylinder Colour Code

	BS 1319–1955 SABS 06–1957	ISO R32	France	
Oxygen	white	white	blanc	white
Nitrous oxide	blue 166	blue	bleu-violet vif	mauve
Cyclopropane	orange 557	orange	orange-gris	orange
Ethylene	violet 796	red	violet	violet
Carbon dioxide	light grey 630	light grey	gris foncé	mid grey
Nitrogen	black	black	noir	black
Helium	mid brown 411	brown	marron foncé	mid brown
Carbogen $(CO_2 + O_2)$	white/grey	white/grey	blanc/bandes gris	white/grey stripes
Entonox $(N_2O + O_2)$	white/blue			
Heliox (He + O_2)	white/brown	white/brown	blanc/bandes marron foncé	
Air	white/black	white/black	noir/bandes blanche	
Vacuum	yellow			
Scavenge	yellow/magenta proposed for ISO standard			
An explosive gas	red			
A poisonous gas	yellow			
Neutral	silver			

27

	USA	Fed. Rep. Germany		DIN 13252
Oxygen	green	blau	blue	(DIN 6164–17:5:2)
Nitrous oxide	blue	grau	grey	(DIN 6164–N:0:3)
Cyclopropane	orange			
Ethylene	red			
Carbon dioxide	grey	schwarz	black	(DIN 6164–N:0:9)
Nitrogen	black			
Helium	brown			
Carbogen (CO_2+O_2)	green/grey			
Entonox (N_2O+O_2)				
Heliox $(He+O_2)$	brown/yellow			
Air	yellow	gelb	yellow	(DIN 6164– 2:6:1)
Oxygen/air		blau/gelb	blue/yellow	(DIN 6164–17:5:2 +2:6:1)
Vacuum		farblos, durchsichtig-clear, transparent		
Scavenge				

Volatile liquid anaesthetic colour code – DIN 13252 Fed. Rep. Germany for bottle to vaporiser indexed couplings:

Halothane	rot	red		
Enflurane	orange	orange		
Methoxyflurane	grün	green		
Trichlorethylene	blau	blue		
Isoflurane	purpur	violet		
Print colours	weiss	white +	schwarz	black
Not allocated	gelb	yellow +	grau	grey

3. Pin Index Code ISO 407

The connecting face of the cylinder is drilled with one or two holes 4.75 mm (0.19 in.) in diameter, to receive mating pins on the yoke assembly. The holes are numbered 1–6 as shown in the first figure, with centres on a radius of 14.3 mm (9/16 in.) as shown in two accompanying figures.

Gas	Index pins
Oxygen	2 and 5
Nitrous oxide	3 and 5
Cyclopropane	3 and 6
Ethylene	1 and 3

Gas	*Index pins*
Carbogen $> 7\%$	1 and 6
Carbogen $< 7\%$	2 and 6
He-Oxygen $> 80\%$	4 and 6
He-Oxygen $< 80\%$	2 and 4
Entonox	Single between 3 and 4
Air	1 and 5

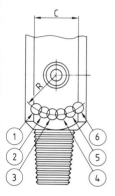

C = 16 mm minimum

R = 14.3 mm nominal

Pin diameter 4 ± 0.1 mm

Pin hole diameter 4.75 mm $\begin{array}{l}+0.1\\-0\end{array}$

Gas delivery socket 7.0 mm $\begin{array}{l}+0.2\\-0\end{array}$

Gas receiving pin 6.5 mm $\begin{array}{l}+0\\-0.2\end{array}$

ISO/R 407-1964(E) + Add. 1-1972

Cylinder value
face with holes

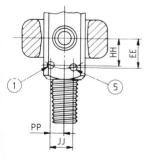

Yoke face
with pins

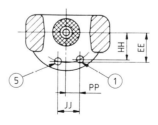

EE	B6	± 0.07 mm	PP	7.15 ± 0.15 mm
HH	12.4	± 0.07 mm	JJ	11.55 ± 0.07 mm

29

4. Cylinder Conversions to Metric Mass

	Existing volume	Mass (g)
Oxygen	300 cu ft	11 520
	270	10 350
	240	9 212
	120	4 606
	48	1 838
	24	930
	12	465
	7	266
Nitrogen	275 cu ft	9 102
	220	7 435
	110	3 717
Air and dry air	275	9 626
	220	7 830
	110	3 915
	150	5 195
	40	1 395
Hydrogen	250 cu ft	602
	210	506
	150	361
	100	241
	162	390
Nitrous oxide	3700 gallons	31 300
	1850	15 600
	200	1 800
	180	1 500
Carbon dioxide	62 lbs	28 200
	31	14 100
	3	1 363
Cyclopropane	35 gallons	284
	20	162
Fumigas 10	64 lbs	2 897
Fumigas 15	64	2 935
Entonox (mass only)		15 430
		7 720
		3 070
		790

5. Conversion Table for Pressures

psi	kPa	atm
1	6.895	0.06805
0.1450	1	9.869×10^{-3}
14.70	101.3	1

6. Solubility of Gases in Water (all at 0°C and 1 atm unless otherwise stated)

Nitrogen	0.023 volumes/volume water
Nitrous oxide	1.3 volumes/volume water
Carbon dioxide	0.759 volumes/volume water
Cyclopropane	0.370 volumes/volume water
Oxygen	0.031 volumes/volume water

7. Purities of Medical Gases

Nitrogen	less than 0.5% oxygen
Nitrous oxide	99.9% minimum
Carbon dioxide	99.0% minimum
Cyclopropane	99.0% minimum
Oxygen	99.5% minimum

G. Flammability Limits of Volatile Anaesthetics

	In air (%)	In oxygen (%)	In nitrous oxide (%)
Diethylether	1.9–48	2.1–82	1.5–24
Divinylether	1.7–27	1.8–85	1.4–25
Ethylchloride	3.8–15.4	4.0–67	2.1–33
Fluroxene	4.2[a]	4.0[a]	4.0[a]
Ethylene	3.1–32	3.0–80	1.9–40
Cyclopropane	2.4–10.4	2.4–63	1.6–30
Chloroform	N.F.	N.F.	N.F.
Trichloroethylene	N.F.	9.0–65	N.F.
Halothane	N.F.	N.F.	above 4.8
Enflurane	N.F.	6	above 5.8
Isoflurane	N.F.	6	above 7.0
Methoxyflurane	9–28[b] above 75 °C	5.2–28[b]	

[a] No upper limit figures have been published

[b] Above clinically used concentrations

H. Saturated Water Vapour Pressures from 0° to 58 °C (mm Hg)

Temp	0	1	2	3	4	5	6	7	8	9
0	4.58	4.92	5.29	5.68	6.09	6.54	7.01	7.51	8.04	8.60
10	9.20	9.83	10.50	11.22	11.97	12.77	13.62	14.51	15.46	16.46
20	17.51	18.63	19.80	21.04	22.35	23.73	25.18	26.71	28.32	30.01
30	31.79	33.66	35.63	37.69	39.86	42.14	44.53	47.03	49.66	52.41

	0	2	4	6	8	10	12	14	16	18
40	55.29	61.46	68.23	75.62	83.69	92.49	102.1	112.5	123.8	136.1

Add temperatures given horizontally to the figure in the left-hand column, e.g., 26.71 mm Hg is for 27°.

Moisture Content of Humid Air

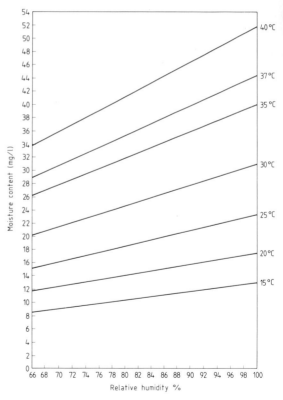

I. Composition of Atmospheric Air

Nitrogen	78.03%	Oxygen	20.99%
Argon	0.93%	Carbon dioxide	0.03%
Neon	0.0015%	Hydrogen	0.001%
Helium	0.0005%	Krypton	0.0001%
Xenon	0.000008%	Smog	Q.S.

Vapour – e.g. water vapour – do not alter the relative composition of air, but reduce the pressure exerted by the gases in the mixture.

J. Atmospheric Pressure

The atmospheric pressure is a general reference level for most biological pressure readings. Such pressures which are measured as a deviation from the atmospheric are termed *gauge pressures* or ATU (AT über). Atmospheric pressure is an *absolute pressure* or ATA (AT absolut).

1 Standard atmosphere = 101.325 kPa = 1.01 Barr = 14.696 psi = 1.0332 kg/cm^2 = 1000 cm H$_2$O = 33.96 ft H$_2$O = 760 mm Hg = 29.92 in. Hg = 760 Torr (mm Hg @ 0 °C) = 1.0581 tons/sq ft.

In the respiratory tract the atmospheric pressure includes the saturated water vapour pressure at 37 °C of 47 mmHg. Anaesthetic vapours are added in a proportion of 1%–5% as a volume/volume ratio.

- At 1500 m (+5000 feet) above sea level pressure is 632 mmHg/84.2 kPa.
- At 3000 m above sea level, pressure is 2/3 that at sea level.
- At 6000 m above sea level, pressure is 1/2 that at sea level.
- At 19000 m above sea level, the atmospheric pressure is equal to water vapour pressure at 37 °C, at which a mammalian body will boil.
- At 10 m under water the ambient pressure is 2 ATA.
- At 20 m under water, at an ambient pressure of 3 ATA and breathing pure oxygen, plasma transfer of oxygen is sufficient to make haemoglobin redundant; acute CNS oxygen toxicity appears.
- At 30 m under water breathing air (4 ATA) nitrogen narcosis is apparent.

K. Species Variations of MAC [5]

	HAL	ENF	ISO	H/E	H/I	I/E
Human being	0.77	1.68	1.15	0.46	0.67	0.68
Rabbit	1.39	2.68	2.05	0.49	0.68	0.72
Cat	1.19	2.37	1.61	0.50	0.74	0.68
Rat (Sprague-Dawley)	1.05	2.21	1.46	0.48	0.72	0.66
Mouse (Swiss-Webster)	0.95	1.95	1.34	0.49	0.71	0.69
Mouse (Charles River)	1.00	2.19	1.41	0.46	0.71	0.64
Dog	0.87	2.06	1.28	0.42	0.68	0.62
Java monkey	1.15	1.84	1.28	0.63	0.90	0.70

HAL: halothane; *ENF:* enflurane; *ISO:* isoflurane; *H/E:* halothane:enflurane; *H/I:* halothane:isoflurane; *I/E:* isoflurane:enflurane

III. Normal Values of Blood Components

A. Normal Blood Biochemical Values

Sodium	133 –146	mmol/l
Potassium	3.5 – 5.5	mmol/l
Calcium – total	2.1 – 2.6	mmol/l
Calcium – ionized	1.14– 1.3	mmol/l
Magnesium	0.75– 1.0	mmol/l
Ammonium (male)	34 – 58	μmol/l
(female)	17 – 51	μmol/l
Chloride	96 –106	mmol/l
Bicarbonate	24 – 30	mmol/l
Phosphate – inorg.	0.8 – 1.4	mmol/l
Sulphate	50 –150	μmol/l
Total fixed base	145 –148	mmol/l
Urea	3.3 – 6.5	mmol/l
Creatinine	60 –120	mmol/l
Uric acid	0.15– 0.6	mmol/l
Glucose	3.0 – 6.0	mmol/l
Total bilirubin	2.5 – 17.0	mmol/l
Direct bilirubin	0 – 6.0	mmol/l
Total protein	60 – 80	g/l
Albumin	35 – 50	g/l
Globulin	20 – 40	g/l
IgG	9.5 – 16.5	g/l
IgA	0.9 – 4.5	g/l
IgM	0.6 – 2.0	g/l
C3	0.94– 2.14	g/l
C4	0.16– 0.5	g/l
Triglyccridcs	0.3 – 1.5	mmol/l
Cholesterol	3.8 – 7.8	mmol/l
Transaminase		
AST or SGOT	0 – 40	μ/l
ALT or SGPT	0 – 53	μ/l
L.D.	100 –350	μ/l
Alkaline phosphatase	30 – 85	μ/l
Osmolality	280 –295	mOsmol/l

B. Moles and Equivalent Weights

Chemical reactions take place between discrete particles of substances, and osmotic pressure is determined by the number of particles in a solution, not by their mass. The **mole** (mol) is the gram molecular mass of a substance; it contains 6.0232×10^{23} particles (Avogadro's constant), using carbon isotope 12 as the reference. Equal volumes of any gas at similar temperature and pressure contain equal numbers of particles, and the gram molecular mass is contained in 22.4 litres at STP. The **millimole** (mmol) is the milligram molecular mass. The **equivalent** (Eq) and **milli-equivalent** (mEq) refers to mass that reacts with a monovalent element. Thus, the equivalent mass of a monovalent element is the same as its atomic mass.

A knowledge of the atomic or molecular mass of elements or simple compounds allows the calculation of equireactive quantities.

Substance/symbol	Atomic mass	Valency	Equivalent mass
Hydrogen – H_2	1 (2)	1	1
Helium – He	4	–	4
Carbon – C	12	4	3
Nitrogen – N_2	14	3/5	
Oxygen – O_2	16	2	8
Fluorine – Fl	19	1	19
Sodium – Na	23	1	23
Magnesium – Mg	24	2	12
Phosphorus – P	31	3	10
Sulphur – S	32	4	8
Chlorine – Cl_2	35	1	35
Potassium – K	39	1	39
Calcium – Ca	40	2	20
Iron – Fe	56	2/3	
Bromine – Br_2	80	1	80
Nitrous oxide – N_2O	44	–	
Carbon dioxide – CO_2	44	–	
Bicarbonate – HCO_3	61	1	61
Carbonate – CO_3	60	2	30
Sulphate – SO_4	96	2	48
Phosphate – PO_4	95	3	32
Dextrose/glucose – $C_6H_{12}O_6$	180	–	180
Urea – N_2H_4CO	60		60

C. Normal Haematological Values

Haematocrit
Adults	47.0 ± 7.0 ml/100 ml
Newborn	44–64 ml/100 ml
Children (varies with age)	35.0–49.0 ml/100 ml

Haemoglobin
Males	16.0 ± 2.0 g/100 ml
Females	14.0 ± 2.0 g/100 ml
Newborn	16.5–19.5 g/100 ml
Children (varies with age)	11.2–16.5 g/100 ml
Fetal	less than 2% total

Cell counts
Erythrocytes
Males	5.4 ± 0.8 million/mm^3
Females	4.8 ± 0.6 million/mm^3
Children (varies with age)	4.5–5.1 million/mm^3

Leucocytes	5000–10 000/mm^3
Myelocytes 0%	0/mm^3
Juvenile neutrophils 3%–5%	150–400/mm^3
Segmented neutrophils 54%–62%	3000–5800/mm^3
Lymphocytes 25%–35%	1500–3000/mm^3
Monocytes 3%–7%	285–500/mm^3
Eosinophils 1%–3%	50–250/mm^3
Basophils 0%–0.75%	15–50/mm^3

(Infants and children have greater relative values)

Platelets	150 000–450 000/mm^3
Reticulocytes	0.5%–1.5% of erythrocytes

Corpuscular values of erythrocytes
(Values are for adults; in children values vary with age)
MCH (mean corpuscular haemoglobin)	29 ± 2.5 pg
MCV (mean corpuscular volume)	87 ± 5 μm^3
MCHC (mean corpuscular haemoglobin concentration)	$34\% \pm 2\%$
MDC (mean cell diameter)	7.5 ± 0.3 μm

Sedimentation rate
Wintrobe
Males	0–6.5 mm in 1 h
Females	0–15 mm in 1 h

Westergren
Males	0–15 mm in 1 h
Females	0–20 mm in 1 h

(may be slightly higher in children and during pregnancy)

D. Normal Coagulation Values

Activated clotting time	80–135 s
Bleeding time (Duke)	1–4 min
Bleeding time (Ivy)	1–6 min
Clot retraction, qualitative	Begins in 30–60 min
Coagulation time (Lee-White)	6–17 min (glass tubes)
Fibrogen, plasma	20–400 mg/100 ml
Fibrinolysins	0
Osmotic fragility of erythrocytes	Begins in 0.45%–0.39% NaCl
Partial thromboplastin time	22–37 s
Prothrombin consumption	Over 80% consumed in 1 h
Prothrombin content	100% (calculated from prothrombin time)
Prothrombin time (one stage)	Same as control (control should be 11–16 s)
Thromboplastin generation test	Compared with normal control
Thrombotest (Owren)	70%–130%

E. Blood Components and Clotting Factors

International nomenclature for clotting factors

Factor	Substance
I	Fibrinogen
II	Prothrombin
III	Tissue thromboplastin
IV	Calcium ions
V	Labile factor
VI	Not assigned
VII	Stable factor
VIII	Antihaemophilic factor (AHF)
IX	Christmas factor
X	Stuart-Power factor
XI	Plasma thromboplastin antecedent (PTA)
XII	Contact factor
XIII	Fibrin-stabilizing factor

The anticoagulant effect of heparin is due to interference in the thrombin fibrinogen reaction and the potentiation of antithrombin III.

Plasma component	*Source of factors*
Fresh-frozen plasma	All coagulation factors – II, V, VII, VIII, IX, X, XI, XII, XIII
Cryoprecipitate (AHF)	Fibrinogen, factors VIII and XIII, von Willebrand's factor
Purified AHF	Factor VIII
Factor IX complex	Factors II, VII, IX, X
Plasma single donor	Stable clotting factors, plasma proteins
Albumin	Pure in 5% and 25% solution
Plasma protein fraction (PPF)	Albumin + alpha and beta globulins 5% solution
Fibrinogen	Sometimes available in dried form
Immune serum globulin	Gamma globulin in 16.5% solution
Rh_o (D) immune globulin	Gamma globulin containing Rh antibodies 15% solution

Other blood products available:

1. Whole blood
   - a) Fresh 24–48 h old
   - b) Standard pack – expires after 28 days
   - c) Paediatric pack
   - d) Leucocyte poor

2. Red cell concentrates (normally HCT 70%)
   - a) Fresh
   - b) Standard
   - c) Washed
   - d) Leucocyte poor
   - e) Frozen
   - f) Adsol, HCT 60%, mannitol, adenine, dextrose

3. Other cells
   - a) Leucocyte concentrate
   - b) Platelet concentrate

F. Oxyhaemoglobin-Dissociation Curves and P Values

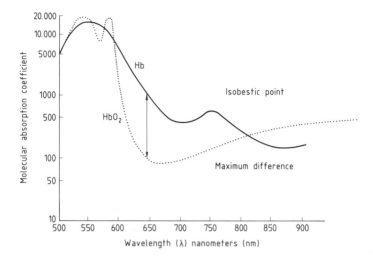

Absorption spectra of reduced (Hb) and oxygenated haemoglobin (HbO_2). The differences in the absorption spectra of oxyhaemoglobin (HbO_2) and reduced haemoglobin (Hb) in visible light are used in the measurement of the degree of oxygen saturation of blood. There are various Isobestic points for these spectra – wavelengths at which absorption by the two pigments is equal. These are at wavelengths 497, 548, 568, 578 and 805 nm. Light absorption at one of these points gives a measure of the total haemoglobin content. Usually the 805 nm point in the infra-red region is used. The maximum difference in the absorption coefficients is at 650 nm in red light, and measurement at this wavelength allows the percentage of HbO_2 in the total Hb to be calculated. Saturation oxymeters may be of the transmission or reflectance type, the latter being preferable when cells are present.

Cyanosis is explained by the ten times greater absorption of red light by Hb than by HbO_2. Hb is both darker and appears more blue-green than HbO_2.

The visible spectrum:

< 400 nm –	ultra-violet	590 nm –	yellow
420 nm –	violet	610 nm –	amber
460 nm –	blue	650–700 nm	red
500 nm –	blue/green	700–740 nm	deep red
550 nm –	green	> 800 nm–	infra-red

The maximum sensitivity of the human eye is for light between ± 500–600 nm in the green to red band. Blue sensitivity is least.

G. Some Causes of Shifts in Oxyhaemoglobin Affinity and Factors That Influence P_{50} [27]

Factors that increase P_{50}	Factors that decrease P_{50}
By direct unknown action	By direct action
Increased temperature	Decreased temperature
Increased (H^+)	Decreased (H^+)
Increased DPG (and ATP)	Decreased pCO_2
Increased Hb concentration	Decreased DPG (and ATP)
Increased ionic strength	Decreased Hb concentration
Abnormal haemoglobin	Decreased ionic strength
Cortisol	Abnormal haemoglobin
Aldosterone	Carboxyhaemoglobin
Pyridoxol phosphate (in Hb solution)	Methaemoglobin
Cell age?	Cell age?
By increasing DPG in cells	By decreasing DPG in cells
Decreased (H^+)	Increased (H^+)
Thyroid hormone	Decreased thyroid hormone
Erythrocytic enzyme deficiency	Erythrocytic enzyme deficiency
Cell age	Cell age
Increased inorganic phosphate	Decreased inorganic phosphate
Inosine	
Increased sulfate	

H. Hypothermia Corrections for pCO_2 and pH

The main confusion arises because the stability of pH-measuring devices depends on constant temperature maintenance. These are kept at 37.5 °C, and thus, above the temperature of the sample when drawn.

1. Optimal function of the cell enzymes is at an offset of $+0.6$ pH units from the neutral point of water, which is pH 7.0 only at 25 °C, and decreases to pH 6.8 at 37.5 °C. Thus normal body pH is 7.4 at normothermia. This offset is maintained constant during cooling by protein buffers.

2. Solubility of carbon dioxide in body fluids increases with cooling, so that the mass dissolved increases if the pCO_2 is constant. In the Henderson-Hasselbach equation that refers to the bicarbonate buffering system, volatile CO_2 is in relation to a fixed mass of sodium in body fluids. To keep the ratio constant requires a lower pCO_2 in blood as temperature falls.

3. If the pH and pCO_2 electrodes are at the same temperature as the hypothermic blood sample, then a raised pH is normal – to 7.6 at 25 °C and a low pCO_2. Hypothermic blood with "normal" pH and pCO_2 values will, on rewarming, show normal values at 37.5 °C. The Kelman and Nunn nomogram has been used to "correct" hypothermic blood samples when measured at normothermia in the belief that a constant pH must be preserved at all temperatures (pHstat technique). This is now no longer regarded as valid. The pH and pCO_2 at other temperatures of a normothermic sample can be derived from this nomogram.

Carbon dioxide solubility in blood increases as body temperature falls by the factors shown, relative to 37° (from Kelman and Nunn [11])

pCO_2	pCO_2
39 °C × 0.9	37 °C × 1
35 °C × 1.09	33 °C × 1.18
31 °C × 1.3	29 °C × 1.41
27 °C × 1.54	25 °C × 1.69
23 °C × 1.85	21 °C × 2.0

Those wishing to attempt their own temperature corrections for pH will have to consider at least the following variables:

1.* The ionization product of water increases with temperature. Only at 24 °C is the pH of neutral water = 7: at 37 °C = 6.8.
2. The pH of some buffers and calibrating solutions used in pH meters varies with temperature.
3. The dissociation constants for plasma protein change.
4. Solubilities of gases increase at low temperatures and can affect body buffers.
5. Boundary effects of glass electrodes may vary and the EMF of the half cells will change.
6. The "ideal" pH for body enzyme systems may vary, and changes in metabolic rate may influence this ideal.

---

* The ion product of water (Kw) at various temperatures (per litre; Pw = pH + pOH):

	Kw	Pw	pH (neutral)
0 °C	0.12×10^{-14}	14.93	7.47
5 °C		14.73	7.37
10 °C	0.29×10^{-14}	14.53	7.27
15 °C	0	14.34	7.17
18 °C	0.59×10^{-14}	14.23	7.11
20 °C		14.166	7.08
24 °C	1.00×10^{-14}	14.00	7.00
25 °C	1.04×10^{-14}	13.996	6.99
30 °C	1.48×10^{-14}	13.83	6.9
35 °C	2.09×10^{-14}	13.68	6.84
40 °C	2.92×10^{-14}	13.53	6.77
50 °C	5.66×10^{-14}	13.26	6.63
60 °C	9.77×10^{-14}	13.01	6.5
100 °C	58.2×10^{-14}	12.24	6.12

To derive the pH of pure water from these figures:

$[H^+]=[OH^-]= \sqrt{Kw}$

At 24 °C $\sqrt{Kw}= \sqrt{10^{-14}} = 10^{-7}$

Thus, $pH=7$

IV. Cardiovascular, Renal, and CSF Values

A. Normal Cardiovascular Values

1. Adults

Blood volume: 5%–7% of body weight in adults
8%–9% of body weight in newborn

Distribution of cardiac output to tissues (as % of cardiac output at rest)

Brain	12% }	
Heart	5% }	Vessel-rich group = 9% of body weight
Kidney	25% }	
Splanchnic bed	25% }	
Muscle and skin	25%	Muscle group = 50% body weight
Fat	5%	Fat ± 19% body weight
Other	8%	Vessel-poor group = 22% body weight
Total	100%	

2. Neonatal

Rate	140/min
Blood volume	85–100 ml/kg
Blood pressure (mean)	56 ± 8 Torr
HCT (%)	54 ± 8
O_2 consumption	6 ml/kg/min

B. The Blood Pressure Cuff

Most non-invasive methods of measuring arterial blood pressure use a blood flow detector distal to an occlusive cuff about the upper arm. Unless this cuff is (a) of **correct size** and (b) **correctly placed,** the pressure within is likely to exceed the occlusive pressure it exerts on the artery, thus leading to false high readings. The midpoint of the cuff must be placed over the brachial artery and be a minimum size in relation to the arm.

WHO recommendation: *Cuff width* should cover approximately 2/3 of the length of the upper arm or be about 20% greater than the diameter of the arm.

Cuff length should be at least 1/2 the circumference of the arm. Dimensions exceeding these mimima do not introduce error, providing the cuff is snugly applied.

Recommended widths:

Leg		Arm	
Adult	15–18 cm	Neonates	2–5 cm
		1–4 years	6 cm
		4–8 years	9 cm
		Adult	12–14 cm

C. Calibrating Intra-arterial Pressure Monitors

Arterial blood pressure is measured by various methods which may not agree because each can measure a slightly different parameter. It has long been known that intra-arterial systolic pressure is higher in the periphery although mean pressures correlate well. This is because there are at least three events during systole that are registered: the initial shock wave on opening of the aortic valve, followed by a rapidly travelling pressure wave, and finally a flow wave. These waves start out of phase and travel at different speeds, and in so doing they further change phase relationships before reaching the periphery. The faster pressure waves may reflect back from the periphery to meet and amplify the slower following waves.

The accuracy of any cannula-catheter-transducer system depends on, inter alia, the natural resonant frequency and its damping, two factors that can be checked.

Natural resonant frequency: If the signal frequencies approach the natural frequency of the measuring system, it will start to resonate with pressure amplification and over-reading. Ideally, the signal frequency should not exceed 66% of the system's natural frequency.

Damping: With sudden pressure changes the pressure measuring system may overshoot and "ring", giving false high peak values. This causes errors in systolic but not diastolic readings. By delaying or damping the response, ringing may be controlled. Three stages of damping of a signal are described:

– Undamped signal – Overshoot is seen even at low frequencies, thus the system overreads and becomes grossly inaccurate at the resonant frequency.

- Critically damped signal – one in which ringing is so well controlled that it cannot fully respond even to low frequency signals. The under-reading error becomes worse as frequency rises.
- Optimally damped signal – responds accurately up to $\pm 65\%$ of the resonant frequency, at which point it starts to tail off.

An underdamped system can be improved by increasing its compliance; in one method a small air bubble is introduced.

Calibrating the Pressure Measuring System

1. Adjust so that the transducer correctly reads static pressure. A 68 cm column of saline (from an unpressurized flushing line) is equivalent to 50 mm mercury.
2. Ringing and the degree of damping can be investigated using the "fast flush" button of an intraflo or similar slow-infusion device to produce a square pressure wave. Set up pressure line and run recorder at 50 mm/s. Briefly pressurize the system, preferably with the downstroke of the square wave falling during diastole so that it is not distorted by the systolic pulse. The resonant frequency is read directly from the trace as the time interval between two pressure peaks as shown in the figure.

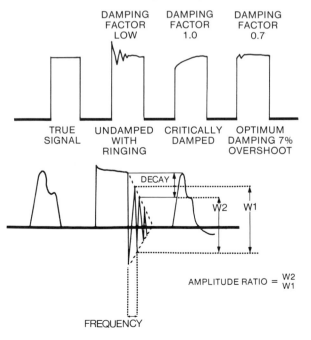

$$\text{Frequency} = \frac{\text{paper speed mm/s}}{\text{one cycle in mm}} \text{ Hz}$$

Damping can be deduced from the rate of decline of the ringing: measure the amplitude of two succeeding waves, and divide the smaller value by the larger. From this the damping factor is obtained from the table (from Gardner [7])

Ratio W2/W1	Damping		Ratio W2/W1	Damping
1	0		0.4	0.28
0.9	0.03		0.3	0.36
0.8	0.075		0.2	0.46
0.7	0.11		0.1	0.6
0.6	0.16		0.05	0.7
0.5	0.22		0.02	0.9

D. Normal Values for Intracardiac Pressures (mmHg)

	Mean	kPa	Range (mmHg)	% O_2 saturation
Central venous pressure (CVP)			4–8	
Right atrium (RA)	5	0–1	1–10	60–70
Right ventricle (RV)	25/5	24/0–1	15–30/0–8	60–70
Pulmonary artery (PA)	23/9	2–4/0.6–2	15–30/5–15	60–70
Pulmonary artery Mean (PAP)	15	2	10–20	
Pulmonary artery wedge pressure (PAWP)	10	0.6–1.7	5–15	100
Left atrium pressure (LA)	8	0.5–1.6	4–12	100
Left ventricular end diastolic pressure (LVEDP)	8		4–12	
Left ventricle (LV)	120/5	12–19/0.5–1.6	120/0–14	97
Aorta	80	12–19/8–12	100–130/70–90	97

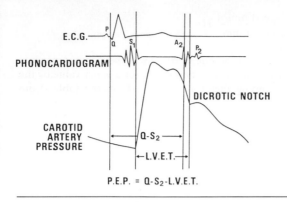

E.C.G.

PHONOCARDIOGRAM

CAROTID
ARTERY
PRESSURE

DICROTIC NOTCH

Q-S₂

L.V.E.T.

P.E.P. = Q-S₂-L.V.E.T.

E. Derived Haemodynamic Parameters

		Adult
CO	$= \mathrm{SV} \times \mathrm{HR}$	5–6 l/min/70 kg
CI	$= \dfrac{\mathrm{CO}}{\mathrm{BSA}}$	3–3.5 l/m²/min
SV	$= \dfrac{\mathrm{CO}}{\mathrm{HR}} \times 1000$	60–90 ml/beat
SI	$= \dfrac{\mathrm{SV}}{\mathrm{BSA}}$	45–60 ml/beat/m²
dp/dt (max)		> 1500 mmHg/s
LVSWI	$= \dfrac{1.36(\overline{\mathrm{MAP}} - \mathrm{PAWP})}{100} \times \mathrm{SI}$	45–60 g m/m²
RVSWI	$= \dfrac{1.36(\overline{\mathrm{PAP}} - \mathrm{PAWP})}{100} \times \mathrm{SI}$	5–10 g m/m²
TPR	$= \dfrac{\overline{\mathrm{MAP}} - \mathrm{CVP}}{\mathrm{CO}} \times 80$	900–1500 dynes/s/cm⁵

		Adult
PVR	$= \dfrac{\overline{PAP} - PAWP}{CO} \times 80$	50–150 dynes/s/cm^5
RPP	$= SP \times HR$	Keep below 12000 in patient with IHS – ischaemic ECG in V5. > 20000, high percentage experience angina
TI	$= SSP \times HR \times PCWP$	Keep < 150000
STI	PEP dp/dt PEP/LVET	$= QS2\text{-}LVET$ $= \dfrac{1}{PEP}$ $= 0.35$ normal
EF	$= \dfrac{ESV - EDV}{EDV}$	$= \dfrac{SV}{EDV} > 0.6$ normal

Abbreviations

BSA	Body surface area
CO	Cardiac output
CVP	Central venous pressure
dp/dt_{max}	Rate of rise of left intraventricular pressure during isometric contraction mmHg/s with normal mitral and aortic valves
EDV	End diastolic volume
EF	Ejection fraction
ESV	End systolic volume
HR	Heart rate
LVET	Left ventricular ejection time
LVSWI	Left ventricular stroke work index
$\overline{MAP}$	Mean systemic arterial pressure
$\overline{PAP}$	Mean pulmonary artery pressure
PAWP	Pulmonary artery wedge pressure
PEP	Pre-ejection period
PVR	Pulmonary vascular resistance
QS_2	Period: Q wave of the ECG to second heart sound
RPP	Mean rate pressure product
RVSWI	Right ventricular stroke work index
SI	Stroke index (usually LV)
SP	Systemic systolic pressure
STI	Systolic time interval
SV	Stroke volume (usually LV)
TI	Triple index
TPR	Total peripheral resistance

F. Renal Function Tests with Normal Values

Clearance Tests:

Inulin clearance (indicates glomerular filtration)	100–150 ml/min
PAH clearance (indicates renal plasma flow)	560–830 ml/min
Creatinine clearance (approximates GFR)	104–125 ml/min
Urea clearance	>70 ml/min
^{51}Cr EDTA (Radioactive technique – blood samples only)	100–150 ml/min

Blood Chemistry:

Osmolality	280	–300	mosmol/kg
Creatinine	8.85–	17.5	mmol/24 h
Sodium	50	–200	mmol/24 h
Urea	2.5 –	7	mmol/l
Urea nitrogen	1.6 –	3.3	mmol/l
Urate (males)	0.15–	0.42	μmol/l
(females)	0.12–	0.39	μmol/l

Indicators of effective excretion

	Sp. Gr.	Osmolality	Urine to plasma ratios		
			Urea	Osmolality	Creatinine
Normal	1000–1040	300–1200	>20:1	>2:1	>100:1
Renal Failure					
Early	1010 fixed	<350	<14:1	<1.7:1	>40:1
Late	1010 fixed	<350	< 5:1	<1.1:1	<25:1
Prerenal Failure	>1022	>400	>20:1	>2:1	>100:1

Oliguria: <0.5 ml/min excretion rate – may be prerenal or renal.

Plasma indicators of acute renal failure:

Increased	potassium*	>7.5 mEq/1
	creatinine	
	fixed acid (metabolic acidosis)*	
	phosphate*	
	urea	>35 mmol/l
	uric acid	
Decreased	Bicarbonate* (metabolic alkalosis)	<15 mmol/l
	calcium	

Sodium and chloride levels are variable.

---

* When the values of the items identified by an asterisk are markedly raised, they are indicators for acute dialysis.

G. Liver Function Tests

Alpha-1-fetoprotein	2–10 µmol/l
Bilirubin	
direct	0–6 mmol/l
indirect	0.2–0.7 mg/100 ml
total	3–20 mmol/l
Bromsulphalein (BSP)	Less that 5% residue in serum 45 min after I.V.I. of 5 mg/kg body weight
Ceruloplasmin	150–600 mg/l
Cholesterol	100–250 mg/100 ml
Cholinesterase	3–8 kU/l (25°)
Enzymes	
Acid phosphatase	0.5–11 iu/l (males)
	0.2–9.5 iu/l (females)
Alkaline phosphatase (ALP)	30–115 iu/l
Amylase	80–180 Somogyi units
Gamma glutamyl transpeptidase (GGT)	15–85 iu/l (males)
	5–55 iu/l (females)
Hydroxybutyrate dehydrogenase (HBD)	100–250 iu/l
Lactate dehydrogenase (LDH)	90–300 iu/l
Aminotransferases	
alanine (ALT)	5–40 iu/l
aspartate (AST)	5–40 iu/l
SGOT	5–40 iu/l
SGPT	5–40 iu/l
Glucose	3.6–6 mmol/l
Proteins	
Albumin	35–50 g/l
Globulin	15–30 g/l
Total	60–80 g/l
Clotting factors	
Prothrombin time	11–13 s
Partial thromboplastin time	32–42 s
Urine bilirubin	nil
Urobilinogen (urine)	0–4 mg/24 h
Urobilinogen (stool)	40–280 mg/24 h

Hepatitis B markers

Marker	Infectivity	
	Low	High
HB$_s$Ag	low titre	high titre
e Antigen	anti-HBe	HBeAg
anti-HBc	low-mid titre	high titre
HBV	absent	present
DNA polymerase	absent	present
Liver Functions	normal	moderately raised

HB$_s$Ag: Hepatitis B surface antigen; HBV: hepatitis B virus; Anti-HB$_c$: hepatitis B core antigen antibody

H. Normal Cerebrospinal Fluid Values

Appearance	Clear, colourless and without clot		
	Child	Adolescent	Adult
Cells: RBC	0–5	at all ages	(mm^3)
Polymorphs	0	presence always	(mm^3)
Lymphocytes	0–5	abnormal at all ages	
Protein	10–20	15–30 10–45	(mg/dl)
Glucose	3.5–4.4	should always be greater than half the blood sugar level	(mmol/l)
Chloride	120–130	at all ages	(mmol/l)
IgG	0.8–6.4		(mg/dl)
Pressure	70–180 mm	water	

Chapter 2

I. Respiratory Parameters

A. Gas Flows in Anaesthetic Circuits (from Mushin and Galloon [20])

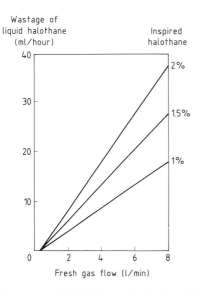

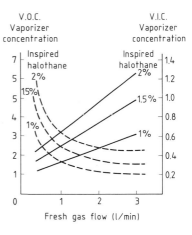

The wastage of liquid halothane related to the fresh-gas flow into the circuit (V.I.C. and V.O.C.). The uptake of halothane by the patient has not been included in this graph, which shows wastage, and not total usage.

Vaporizer concentrations required to obtain inspired concentrations of 1, 1.5 and 2 per cent with the V.I.C. and the V.O.C., with various fresh-gas flows. With the V.O.C. high vaporizer concentrations are needed, with the V.I.C. only low ones are necessary.

1. Systems in Which No Rebreathing is Possible
Fresh gas flow (FGF) is set to patient's ventilation requirements.

2. Systems in Which Rebreathing is Possible

(a) Magill System

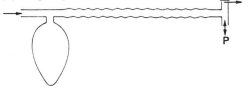

Minimal fresh gas delivery must never fall below alveolar minute ventilation, and should be preferably 50% higher.
- Spontaneous ventilation – gas flow equal to *total* minute volume in adults
- Controlled ventilation – gas flow $2.5 \times$ total minute volume
- Apparatus dead space too large for children
- More efficient with spontaneous than controlled ventilation
- Preferred flow for spontaneous ventilation: 70 ml/kg/min FGF

(b) Bain System

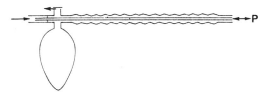

- Spontaneous ventilation: 150–200 ml/kg/min FGF
- Controlled ventilation: at $pCO_2 \pm 40$ Torr – 70 ml/kg/min FGF
                               at $pCO_2 \pm 32$ Torr – 100 ml/kg/min FGF
- Low dead space makes circuit suitable for children.
- Neonates 3 l/min at 40 b.p.m. and TV 10 ml/kg

(c) Ayre's T-piece

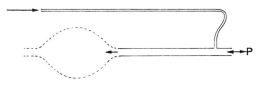

- Spontaneous ventilation: 200 ml/kg body weight or 3 × minute volume
- Controlled ventilation: as for Bain circuit
- Bain and Ayre are similar circuits; Ayre is more efficient, since external supply tube improves plug flow in expiratory limb.

(d) Rebreathing Systems with Soda Lime

(systems in which rebreathing is intended)
All such systems use soda lime for expired carbon dioxide adsorption.

There are two configurations:
- To-and-fro movement of respired gas through a soda lime canister close to patient; no unidirectional valves
- Circulating (circle) system, in which respired gas passes through soda lime canister remote from patient through unidirectional valves

These circuits can be used with gas flows similar to those in the Bain and Magill systems, down to flows equal to basal uptake. Details of technique with very low flows are given in next section.

Anaesthetic vaporizers should be used *outside* the breathing circuit (VOC) to avoid water condensation and inadvertent overdose, as inspired concentration is always less than that delivered by vaporizer.

(e) Apparatus Dead Space

Any apparatus dead space which becomes an extension of the anatomical dead space leads to lower FIO_2 and higher $FICO_2$ than are delivered by the gas source.

"Apparatus dead space" is any space within which there is pure to-and-fro movement of respiratory gases without addition or removal of constituents. In circuits without soda lime, fresh gas flow can greatly influence the effective size of apparatus dead space by replacing to-and-fro movement with unidirectional flow.

B. Low-Flow Anaesthetic Techniques

Definition: The use of fresh gas flows (FGF) of less than 3 litres/min into an adult breathing system. Such low flows necessitate the rebreathing of expired gas, possible only with carbon dioxide absorption and oxygen enrichment.

Disadvantages: The more the minute respiratory volume exceeds the FGF, the greater the difference between the composition of FGF and inspired air, such that soluble components decrease.

Standard vaporizers do not deliver adequate induction concentrations at low flows; the mass vaporized per minute is too small.

Advantages: Large internal volume with low FGF stabilizes inspired gas composition, and contains large oxygen reserve.

Economy – consumption *can* be reduced tenfold over longer operation. Humidity is maintained at about 50%.

A totally closed system allows measurement of uptake of oxygen and anaesthetics, CO_2 production, FRC, etc.

Essentials: Leak-proof breathing system with oxygen analyser, rising bellows ventilator (no subatmospheric pressure), high output vaporizers or liquid injection. Volatile agent analyser is needed with totally closed circuit.

Techniques: Usually, a high initial gas flow for denitrogenation and to cover rapid uptake phase. Oxygen analyser has value in nitrous oxide-based techniques. Technique may then be either totally closed, or low flow with leak. Advisable to use high flow for a short period each hour and after any circuit disconnection to wash out nitrogen.

1. Pre-oxygenation/denitrogenation followed by 100% nitrous oxide ± 1 l/min and halothane until oxygen analyser reaches 30% when oxygen is reintroduced. Maintain constant and expired volume with N_2O or O_2 with closed system (Hershey technique).
2. Pre-oxygenation followed by volatile agent in oxygen. At basal oxygen flows of ± 200 ml/min no standard vaporizer can input sufficient mass for induction. Use liquid injection, two or three vaporizers in series, or veterinary vaporizer with analyser.
3. Entonox at FGF of 1 l/min (50% $O_2 + N_2O$) gives stable PiO_2 between 30%–40% after induction, since uptake of oxygen is greater than of nitrous oxide. Halothane supplement is possible with standard vaporizer (Glasgow technique).

4. After initial 15-min induction period, select a low flow of gas/oxygen mixture (750/250) and add to this the predicted minute uptake of each ($\pm 150 + 200$) to give a total flow of about 1000/500. This flow being about 4–5 times the uptake rate, circuit composition is stable. Input of 1% halothane gives 0.6%–0.7%. Alternatively, use system of Virtue, with 200 ml $O_2 + 300$ ml N_2O to give 20%–40% O_2 (use O_2 analyser).

Using Liquid Anaesthetic Agent Injection: This presents a conceptual problem to anaesthetists accustomed to equilibrating a patient against a chosen concentration. Liquid injection into a closed circuit is equivalent to the i. v. injection of a dose calculated from pharmakokinetic models, unless a vapour analyser is used. Rate of uptake is roughly inversely proportional to the square root of time in minutes from start. Details of method may be found in Lowe and Ernst [17].

Principles:
1. Use 1-ml all-glass syringe for liquid injection through T connection with tap into breathing circuit. (Take care to avoid accidental i. v. injection.)
2. All volatile agents produce ± 200 ml vapour per 1 ml liquid (see Table 1).
3. Unless micro-injection techniques are used, only inject liquid bolus into the expiratory limb of a circle absorber to avoid high concentration peaks.
4. Requirements for a given application:
   - **System Prime** - a liquid bolus before start of anaesthesia to achieve a suitable starting concentration (e. g. 1.3 MAC) in a compartment comprising:
     - - Breathing circuit (± 50 dl)
     - - Patient FRC (calculated as 0.3 dl/kg)
     - - Minute carriage in arterial blood (minute cardiac output $\pm 2 \times kg^{0.75}$).

Table 1. For 0.65 MAC volatile agent

Agent	ml vapour/ ml liquid @ 37°C	Liquid anaesthetic dose (L) and prime dose (P)												
		40 kg		50 kg		60 kg		70 kg		80 kg		90 kg		100 kg	
		L	P	L	P	L	P	L	P	L	P	L	P	L	P
Halothane	240	0.6	0.3	0.7		0.4	0.8 0.4	0.9	0.5	1.0	0.5	1.1	.57	1.2	0.6
Enflurane	210	1.3	0.6	1.5		0.8	1.7 0.9	2.0	1.0	2.1	1.1	2.3	1.2	2.5	1.3
Isoflurane	206	0.8	0.4	0.9		0.5	1.0 0.5	1.2	0.6	1.3	0.6	1.4	0.7	1.6	0.8
Diethylether	246							7.1						10.0	

- **Liquid Dose Unit** – this is the minute transport of agent by arterial blood during the first minute, or the amount to be added to maintain the prime concentration. It is calculated as 2 × minute arterial delivery – (cardiac output × solubility × concentration).
- **Time Units** – it is easier to use a fixed volume and to inject it over progressively longer time periods as anaesthesia progresses. The first time period is 1 min; thereafter the volume injected per minute decreases according to $1/t^{0.5}$, or a constant volume is injected over periods $t^{0.5}$ (see Table 2).
- **Concentration Goals** – with a pure oxygen inhalation technique 1.3 MAC is used; with nitrous oxide at 65%, 0.65 MAC is target concentration

Table 2. Time units in which liquid dose unit is injected (min)

Time unit	1 (+2)	3 (+2)	5 (+2)	7 (+2)	9 (+2)	11 (+2)	13
Elapsed time	1	4	9	16	25	36	49

C. Capnography

By the use of a rapid-response CO_2 analyser, the end-expired pCO_2 can be followed. Normal trace exhibits typical end-expiratory plateau at a pCO_2 similar to arterial levels.

Causes of Decreased End-expired pCO_2

1. Hyperventilation
2. Inadequate sampling volume
3. Incorrect placement of sampling catheter (in fresh gas stream)
4. Hypothermia
5. Incipient pulmonary oedema
6. Air embolism
7. Decreased blood flow to lungs: shock – cardiac arrest – hypotension

Causes of Increased End-expired pCO$_2$

1. Hypoventilation
2. NaHCO$_3$ infusion
3. Laparoscopy (CO$_2$ inflation)
4. Anaesthetic breathing circuit error:
   Inadequate fresh gas flow
   Rebreathing
   Faulty circle absorber valves
   Exhausted soda lime
5. Hyperthermia – malignant hyperthermia
6. Improved blood flow to lungs – following resuscitation, after hypotension
7. Water in capnograph head

Causes of Abnormal Wave Form

1. Partial curarisation
2. Poor intrapulmonary gas mixing
3. Technical errors

D. Simple Pulmonary Function Values

	Ages 16–34		Ages 35–49		Ages 50–69	
	Women	Men	Women	Men	Women	Men
Vital capacity (supine; l)	2.3–4.2	2.8–5.0	2.2–3.4	3.2–5.2	1.6–3.5	2.2–5.4
FEV$_1$ (standing; l)	2.0–3.7	2.4–4.4	1.9–2.9	2.7–4.4	1.3–2.8	1.8–4.4
FEV$_1$ (% VC)	87 ± 5		84 ± 6		81 ± 5	
Maximum Breathing Capacity (standing; l/min)	60–120	80–170	50–110	90–140	50–100	60–140
O$_2$ consumption (ml/min/m^2 BSA)	110–150	130–180	110–135	120–160	105–150	110–165
Functional Residual Capacity (supine; l)	2.15	2.0	2.0	1.9	1.9	1.7

E. Pulmonary Function Tests*

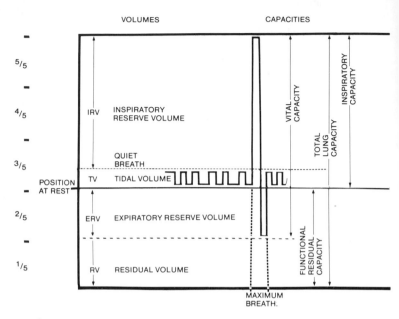

THE $1/5$ UNITS VARY BETWEEN 1 LITRE – 1.25 LITRE IN AVERAGE ADULTS.

THE POSITION AT REST POINT INCREASES WITH AGE.

THERE ARE 4 VOLUMES THAT DO NOT OVERLAP

CAPACITIES ARE COMBINATIONS OF VOLUMES.

1. Lung Volumes – Prediction Formulae:

	Adult male equations	Adult female equations
FVC (forced vital capacity)	$0.065 \times H_{cm} - 0.029 \times A - 5.459$	$0.037 \times H_{cm} - 0.22 \times A - 1.774$
TLC (total lung capacity)	$0.094 \times H_{cm} - 0.015 \times A - 9.17$	$0.078 \times H_{cm} - 0.01 \times A - 7.36$
FRC (functional residual capacity)	$0.0508 \times H_{cm} - 5.159$	$0.047 \times H_{cm} - 4.854$

---

* Authored by C. M. Lewis

In normal subjects 50% FRC = RV (residual volume) = ERV (expiratory reserve volume). The above predictions are for the erect posture. In the supine position, FRC reduces by 16%–25%, i.e. by one-sixth to one-quarter, due to ERV reduction.

RV/TLC is normally 20%–25%, but may increase to 40% in old age or with emphysema.

FEV_1/FVC exceeds 69% where there is normal airflow, but falls in obstructive airway disease. Exceptionally high values are seen in restrictive lung disease.

The area under the flow-volume curve (AFV_E) may be predicted from the equation

$$0.049 \times PEFR \text{ (peak expiratory flow rate)} \times FVC$$

It is an extremely sensitive screening measurement; values below 70% of predicted indicate lung function abnormality due to ventilatory restriction or airflow obstruction, where as all or most other indices still indicate normality.

2. Interpretation for Diagnosis:

The normal range for lung volumes is taken as 80%–120% predicted: this covers $2 \times SD$ on a normal population distribution, i.e. 95% of normal subjects will fall into this range.

Airflow obstruction is present and is

	FEV_1/FVC	AFV_E
Mild, where	61%–69%	41%–69%
Moderate, where	45%–60%	25%–40%
Severe, where	less than 45%	less than 25% of predicted values

Restrictive abnormality is present when TLC and vital capacity (where airflow is normal) are reduced, and is ...

Mild, where both indices fall	between 66% and 80% of predicted
Moderate	between 51% and 65%
Severe	below 50% of predicted normal values

3. Intrapulmonary Gas Mixing

Normal values for the alveolar slope (phase III) of the single-breath O_2 nitrogen washout curve in N_2% change/l are 1.2% at age 20, increasing linearly to 2.7% at age 60. For smokers the linear increase is to 4.5% at age 60.

An increased slope indicates an impaired intrapulmonary gas distribution, poor mixing, regional inhomogeneities, compliance differences, and airway closure encroaching on tidal volume by exceeding FRC.

4. "Ideal" Alveolar PO$_2$ and Alveolar-Arterial Oxygen Gradient:

$$PAO_2 = (P_B - PH_2O)(FIO_2) - PaCO_2/R$$
$$= 713 (FIO_2) - 1.25 \cdot PaCO_2$$

$P(A-aDO_2) = PAO_2 - PaO_2$, or (roughly, where cardiac output is normal and no COPD)

$$= 145 - (PaO_2 + PaCO_2)$$

At $FIO_2 = 0.21$ normal is $10-20$ mmHg, or $2.5 + (age \times 0.21)$, while PaO_2 (mmHg) may be predicted from $104.2 - (age \times 0.27)$. At $FIO_2 = 0.21$ the A-aDO$_2$ reflects anatomical shunt plus V_A/Q inequality (physiological or functional shunt).

A-aDO$_2$ on oxygen is usually under 30 mmHg in young subjects, but is up to 60 mmHg at ages 60–70.

5. Shunt Equations:

1. $$\frac{Q_S}{Q} = \frac{CcO_2 - CaO_2}{CcO_2 - CvO_2}$$

(CcO$_2$ is derived from PAO$_2$ and the appropriate temperature and acid-base corrected oxyhaemoglobin-dissociation curve).

At $FIO_2 = 0.21$ this measures total pulmonary-venous admixture (anatomical shunt plus V_A/Q inequality).

2. At FIO_2 greater than 0.40 the Ayres simplification may be used:

$$\frac{Q_S}{Q_T} = \frac{(PAO_2 - PaO_2) \cdot 0.0031}{(CaO_2 - CvO_2) + (PAO_2 - PaO_2) \cdot 0.0031}$$

This measures only true pathological and anatomical shunting, not the functional shunt of V_A/Q inequality (venous admixture effect).

Note:

Both A-aO$_2$ and shunt fractions are influenced by Q_T and haemoglobin. A low cardiac output with high $(C(a-\bar{v})O_2$ yields a low PaO$_2$ with increased A$_0$aDO$_2$ and Q_{ps}/Q_T (physiological shunt).

6. Dead Space Equation (Bohr):

$$\frac{V_D}{V_T} = PaCO_2 = \frac{P_ECO_2}{PaCO}$$

This is normally 0.3 at rest. In seated normal subjects $V_D/V_T\%$ may be predicted from $24.6 + 0.17 \times$ age (years)

Anatomical dead space may be estimated as mass (kg) $\times 2.2$ in ml. Alveolar dead space = physiological dead space − anatomical dead space, or may be derived directly from:

$$\frac{a - ET\ DCO_2}{PaCO_2} \cdot V_t$$

7. Oxygen Flux or Availability (Nunn):

$$O_2\ flux = Q_T\ CaO_2$$
$$= \text{cardiac output } \frac{HbO_2\ saturation\%}{100} \times Hb\ (g/dl) \times 1.34$$

The normal value exceeds 100.

F. Flow Volume Curves

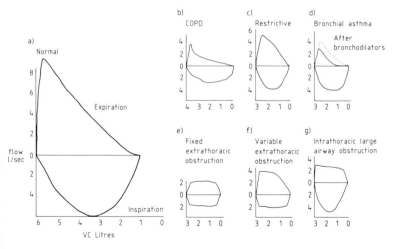

G. Some Clinical Tests of Respiratory Function

The following tests are rough indicators of pulmonary pathology that are of value where laboratory facilities are unavailable. They are grouped according to the main parameter examined and roughly graded into normal, significantly abnormal, and seriously abnormal.

Accurate assessment should not be expected from any one test. By comparing the results of several tests, by noting the effect of bronchodilators, and by following daily serial measurements, valuable clinical information on the progress of disease can be obtained.

(A) Expiratory Flow Rate

1. Auscultate over the L lung base during forced expired vital capacity. Time the duration of normal alveolar breath sounds.

Normal	2 s
Significant	2-6 s
Serious	6 s

   Seriously compromised function may not allow expiratory breath holding beyond 6 s. Do not read adventitious sounds for vesicular sounds.
2. The Bag Pipe Sign: The continuation of adventitious sounds (wheezes, rales, etc.) after the end of expiratory flow indicates an $FEV_1 < 30\%$.
3. Cough effectiveness in the absence of pain: In adults inability to clear loose secretion usually signifies an FEV_1 of < 1 litre ($\mp 25\%$ VC). This figure applies to obstructive lung disease, not to restrictive disease where effective coughing is still present at low lung volumes.

(B) Peak Flow

1. Blow out a burning match through open lips:

Normal	beyond 15 cm
Significant	10-15 cm
Severe	below 10 cm

2. Wright's Peak Flow Meter:

Normal	above 300 l/min
Significant	below 150 l/min
Severe	below 100 l/min

   There are large variations in peak flows depending on age, sex and body stature.

(C) Maximal Force of Respiratory Muscles

1. Expiratory Force: Blow up a sphygmomanometer column and hold the pressure for 5 s.

   Normal   above 150 mmHg
   Significant   below 100 mmHg

   The force generated gives a measure of cough effectiveness. Since this is a Valsalva manoeuvre, it can also indicate circulatory pathology if the blood pressure is followed. The ability to maintain a normal or raised BP in the presence of raised intrathoracic pressure for > 20 s may indicate cardiac failure with increased central blood volume. Unstable blood pressure indicates hypovolaemia.

2. Inspiratory Force: Inspiration from the resting end expiratory position against a mercury column holding the peak negative pressure for 5 s.

   Normal   30 mmHg
   Significant   20 mmHg
   Severe   10 mmHg

(D) Ventilation Volumes

1. Circumferential chest expansion from full expiration to full inspiration measured at the "nipple line" (insurance company tests).

   Normal   5–7 cm minimum
   Significant   2–4
   Severe < 2

   Chest movement related to diaphragmatic (abdominal) movement is an important differentiator between restrictive and obstructive disease.

2. Wright's Respirometer can record the various static ventilatory volumes. Vital capacity is roughly predicted on the basis of formula on page 49.

(E) Ventilation and Gas exchange

1. Measure minute volume using Wright's Respirometer or equivalent. Extrapolate from volume and frequency over 15 s or measure volume over 1 min.

   Relate to Ventilation Nomogram on page 69 (Vb)

   Normal   5–8 l/min

   Both ventilatory and haemodynamic factors are involved.

   Raised minute volume may indicate raised V_d/V_t, or increased metabolic needs as in fever. Lowered minute volume indicates ventilatory failure or respiratory centre depression (CO_2, drugs, disease, hypoxia).

2. Inspiratory/expiratory ratios:

Normal	$1:2$ with passive end expiratory pause
Significant	$>1:4$ with active end of expiration
	$>1:4$ with active expiration indicates gas exchange defect or increased metabolic need

3. Breath-Holding Test. Holding breath in full inspiration.

| Normal | 1 min |
| Significant | 30 s |

(F) Closing Volume

1. With the patient standing during slow expiration from full inspiration, auscultate over the trachea for onset of end expiratory wheeze; measure the vital capacity with a respirometer and relate this to the volume at onset of wheezing.

   Normal– wheeze after 80% expiration

   Significant– wheeze between 40% and 80% expiration

   Severe – wheeze at 40% or less expiration

   These figures can be of some significance only in the absence of active bronchospasm.

(G) Other Clinical Signs

1. Nail bed/mucous membrane cyanosis – indicates severe disturbance
2. Movement of alae nasi
3. Recession of intercostal muscles
4. Activity of accessory respiratory muscles
5. Warm periphery and rapid capillary refill with cyanosis – indicates CO_2 retention in respiratory failure
6. Response to exercise with dyspnoea before significant tachycardia (120 bpm)
7. Pursed-lip, breathing on expiration indicates large airway instability – anticipate problems with intubation, consider PEEP
8. Hoover's sign – indrawing of lower costal margins during inspiration – indicates positive transpulmonary pressure (i.e. over distension of the lung as in severe emphysema)
9. Inability to complete a sentence in one breath
10. Haemoglobin 17-18 g% – indicates chronic hypoxaemia

H. Normal Neonatal Values

Respiratory:

Rate (f)	30–40/min
Minute ventilation (VE)	100–150 ml/kg/min
Wasted ventilation (VD)	2 ml/kg
Tidal volume (VT)	7 ml/kg
PO_2	50 Torr
PCO_2	30 Torr

I. Radford's Ventilation Nomogram

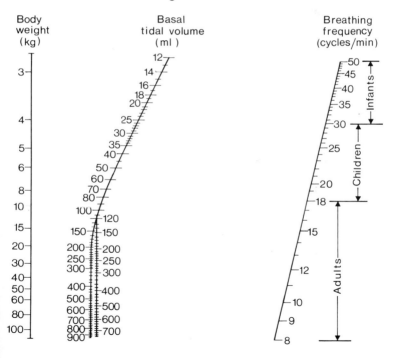

Body weight (kg) — Basal tidal volume (ml) — Breathing frequency (cycles/min)

To allow the incorporation of Radford's Ventilation Nomogram [24] into computer programmes, horizontal lines may be drawn across it mathematically connecting body weight with tidal volume and frequency, using the formulae:

(1) $Y = A + B \times X$

where Y = predicted tidal volume
        $A = 2.7476$
        $B = 8.0306$
        X = body weight

(2) $Y = A + B/X$

where Y = breathing frequency for the tidal volume
        $A = 7.5393$
        $B = 103.2556$
        X = body weight

Corrections which are to be applied mathematically:

- Fever: add 9% for each degree centigrade above 38°
- Altitude: add 8% for each 1000 m above sea level
- Endotracheal intubation: subtract a volume in cc equal to the body weight in kg
- Metabolic acidosis: requires compensatory hyperventilation of 20% if base deficit > 5
  Breathing circuits: add volume equal to the dead space.

J. Blood Gas Parameters in Various Acid-Base Disturbances (Henderson-Hasselbach)

	pH	$PaCO_2$	HCO_3	CO_2 content	Base excess
Normal values	7.35–7.45	35–45 Torr 4.6–6.0 kPa	24–26 mEq/l	25–28 mEq/l	± 3 mEq/l
Metabolic acidosis	↓	↓	↓	↓	↓
Acute respiratory acidosis	↓	↑	↔	slight ↑	↔
Compensated respiratory acidosis	↔ or slight ↓	↑	↑	↑	↔
Metabolic alkalosis	↑	slight ↑	↑	↑	↑
Acute respiratory alkalosis	↑	↑	↔	slight ↓	↔
Compensated respiratory alkalosis	↔ or slight ↑	↓	↓	↓	↔

K. Correction of Metabolic Acidosis Based upon Base Excess and Body Weight

Base excess of $+5$ mEq/l to -5 mEq/l will normally be corrected without treatment.

When base deficit is found to exceed 5 mEq/l the volume of bicarbonate necessary for correction is calculated:

Base deficit in mEq/l × body weight in kg × 0.3

The standard sodium bicarbonate solutions contain:

$NaHCO_3$ 8.4% = 1 mEq/ml
$NaHCO_3$ 4.2% = 0.5 mEq/ml

The factor of 0.3 reflects the extracellular fluid volume in which the H^+ to be buffered by sodium solutions is largely distributed.

Total body water in litres is 0.6 × body weight in kg.

Two regimes are advocated for metabolic acidosis correction:

1. Calculate dose necessary to correct base excess to 0 mEq/l; give half calculated dose; recheck base excess and serum sodium values before administering further bicarbonate.
2. On the assumption that a base excess of up to $+5$ mEq/l is acceptable, the full calculated correction dose can be given, provided serum sodium is not abnormally raised.

The intrinsic ability of the body to correct metabolic acidosis depends on:

- Adequate oxygenation
- Adequate carbohydrate substrate
- Adequate tissue perfusion
- Normal body temperature
- Adequate renal function

L. Oxygen Delivery to Tissues

Delivery of oxygen by the blood to tissue beds depends on:

a) Cardiac output
b) Haemoglobin concentration
c) Oxygen saturation of haemoglobin

Normal adult values:

Cardiac output	± 5 l/min
Haemoglobin	12–14 g%
Oxygen binding	1.39 ml O_2 per 1 g Hb
Oxygen saturation	100%

Normal carrying capacity for oxygen is thus in the region of 20 ml/100 ml blood, and normal tissue delivery is 5 ml/100 ml blood, of which up to 10 ml/100 ml can be delivered before tissue hypoxia becomes serious (see Oxyhaemoglobin-dissociation curves).

Oxygen delivery may be prejudiced by:

a) Low cardiac output (shock, heart failure)
b) Anaemia
c) Too rapid passage of blood through the lungs
d) Other general causes of hypoxaemia
e) Peripheral vasoconstriction

Table: Tissue oxygen stores (70 kg adult)

Volume	Breathing air	Breathing oxygen
In the lungs (FRC)	450 ml	3000 ml
In the lungs (VC)*	1200 ml	6000 ml
Carried in blood	850 ml	950 ml
Tissue fluids	50 ml	100 ml
Bound to myoglobin	200 ml	200 ml
Total at FRC	1550 ml	4250 ml
Total at VC	2300 ml	7250 ml

* At peak breath holding

Preoxygenation thus makes about 2500 ml of extra oxygen available, or enough to cover a period of apnoea lasting roughly 10 min.

The quantity of oxygen in physical solution in tissue fluids is 0.0225 ml/dl/kPa at 37 °C. At sea level with air breathing this represents about 0.3 ml/dl (note: alveolar $pO_2 = 13$ kPa) and 2.3 ml/dl whilst breathing 100% oxygen. Myoglobin saturates at low partial pressure – P_{50} is 0.4 kPa as against 3.6 kPa for haemoglobin.

M. Reading a Chest X-Ray

PA or AP view: indicates tube to film direction
Lateral view: side nearest film indicated

A. General

Correct patient?	Date
Penetration	Inspiration/expiration
Standing/sitting/supine	Trachea central
Sex – breast shadows	Surgical emphysema
Stomach air bubble	Foreign bodies

B. Boundaries

Ribs	Fractures
	Angle to spine
	Other pathology
Diaphragm	Curvature
	Distortion
	Flattening/paralysis
	Air under diaphragm
Mediastinum	Width, lateral shift
	Tracheal bifurcation

C. Heart

Size	Ratio of heart width to transverse diameter at diaphragm level

Lateral borders defined:

Right border	Right atrium
	Hilar vessels
	Right ventricle
Left border	Aortic knuckle
	Left atrium
	Hilar vessels
	Left ventricle

D. Lungs

	Density increase/decrease, apex to base
	Volume (no. of ribs) emphysema
	Hilum displaced
	Costophrenic angles
	L and R interlobar fissures, position, fluid
	Collapse left lower lobe
	Pneumothorax
	Pleural thickening
Parenchyma	Density: compare L and R apices, mid-zones, bases
	Signs of oedema
	Localized lesion
	Diffuse lesions – "snowstorm"
	Tumours – hilar glands
	Lung vessels – ? reversed flow
	Air bronchogram

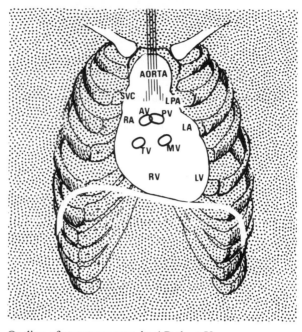

Outline of structures seen in AP chest X-ray

SVC: Superior vena cava; *RA:* right atrium; *RV:* right ventricle; *LV:* left ventricle; *LA:* left atrium; LPA: left pulmonary artery; *AV:* aortic valve; PV: pulmonary valve; *TV:* tricuspid valve; *MV:* mitral valve

75

II. Respiratory Assessment and Support

A. Indications and Contraindications for Endotracheal Intubation

Specific Anaesthetic Indications for Endotracheal Intubation

1. Operations where a free airway is compromised or cannot otherwise be maintained
2. In patients who may have a full stomach or incompetent gastro-oesophageal junction
3. All intrathoracic and intra-abdominal cases under general anaesthesia
4. Following the use of long-acting muscle relaxants
5. Operations on the head and neck
6. Paediatric anaesthesia (to reduce dead space)
7. Where laryngeal spasm is likely to develop
8. Paralysis of the vocal cords

Contraindications

1. Acute laryngitis or tracheitis
2. Malignancies of larynx (seeding of cells into tracheobronchial tree)
3. Allergy to endotracheal tube materials
4. Aneurysm of aortic arch
5. Open pulmonary tuberculosis

Difficulty with Intubation

1. A short muscular neck and a full set of teeth
2. A receding lower jaw or prominent premaxilla
3. A high arched palate
4. Protruding upper incisors, absent incisors
5. Difficulty in opening jaw, including arthritis
6. Contractures of neck tissues
7. Arthritis of cervical spine
8. Haematomata, abscesses and tumours of the pharynx and larynx
9. Arthritic fixation of laryngeal joints
10. High transverse ridge in nasopharynx – nasal intubation

Complications

(A) At Intubation

1. Trauma	– lips, teeth	
	– retropharyngeal dissection	
	– aspiration	
	– oesophageal intubation	
	– endobronchial intubation	
2. Reflex	– laryngovagal	– bradycardia or arrest
	– laryngosympathetic	– tachycardia, ventricular extra-systole
	– laryngospinal	– coughing
		– vomiting
	– bronchospasm	

3. Pharmacomechanical:

- increased intraocular pressure
- hypotension
- bronchospasm and other allergy
- raised intracranial pressure

(B) After Intubation

1. Respiratory obstruction
2. Haemorrhage
3. Ruptured "cuff"
4. Aspiration
5. Bronchospasm

(C) At Extubation

1. Failure to remove accumulated secretions
2. Trauma   – glottis when cuff inflated
                 – tracheal mucosa
                 – laryngospasm
                 – glottic oedema

Indications for Awake Intubation

1. Upper airway obstruction
2. Anatomical and pathological conditions that may make intubation difficult
3. Poor risk case – allows slow induction of anaesthesia
4. Respiratory failure
5. Full stomach
6. Premature baby or neonate
7. Pierre-Robin Syndrome

Methods

1. Superior laryngeal nerve block
2. Local spray
3. Transtracheal analgesia
4. Glossopharyngeal block
5. Nerve block through thyrohyoid membrane

B. Pre- and Postoperative Respiratory Considerations

Dyspnoea grade	Suggested preoperative test*
I. Normal	None
II. Abnormal, but walks unlimited distance in own time	Spirometry;** × chest X-ray; EKG; HCT
III. Specific limitation on level walking, e.g. 2–3 blocks	Spirometry, arterial blood gases if spirometry abnormal; EKG; chest X-ray; HCT
IV. Dyspnoea on limited exertion	Spirometry; gases; EKG; chest X-ray; HCT
V. Dyspnoea at rest	Spirometry poorly tolerated; gases, EKG, chest X-ray, HCT

Likelihood and severity of postoperative respiratory complications	Anticipated need for postoperative respiratory intervention
I. Infrequent	Minimal
II. Infrequent for extremity and lower abdominal surgery; more likely with thoracic and upper abdominal	Unlikely, but should be observed closely
III. Infrequent with extremity surgery; common with abdominal and thoracic surgery	For abdominal and thoracic surgery, extubation only after careful PAR evaluation; may need ventilation
IV. High frequency except with short peripheral procedures	May require ventilation for some hours or longer
V. Very high; only essential surgery should be done.	As for IV

* Tests which characterize disorders and check impression gained from dyspnoea history
** Vital capacity, FEV

C. Indications for Respiratory Support

1. Pre-existing lung disease with signs of ventilatory failure:
   a) Adult respiratory rate $> 40/\text{min}$
   b) $V_D/V_T > 0.6$
   c) $PaCO_2 > 50$ Torr
   d) $PaO_2 < 60$ Torr
   e) $A - a\ DO_2 > 300$ Torr when $FIO_2 = 1$
   f) $VC < 15$ ml/kg body mass
   g) $FEV_1 < 45\%$
2. Depression of respiratory centre by drugs, disease or injury
3. Chest wall injury which includes surgery of the chest wall
4. (Incipient) pulmonary oedema and respiratory distress syndrome
5. Open pneumothorax
6. To relieve patient of the metabolic load of the work of breathing
7. Obesity – especially pickwickian syndrome
8. Upper abdominal surgery, especially in patients who are old, obese, or have abdominal distension
9. Shock, fat embolism
10. After cardiac arrest
11. For the control of secretions and the prevention of aspiration
12. Massive blood transfusion, especially without 20–40 μm filter
13. Hypothermia below 30 °C
14. Diseases of muscle and neuromuscular junction – abnormal reaction to relaxants
15. As part of an effective pain control regime using opiates
16. For control of intracranial pressure

D. Criteria for Weaning from Respirator

Criteria are based upon the effectiveness of ventilatory function and the general condition of the subject. In many respects they are the converse of those upon which controlled ventilation is instituted.

1. Sequential monitoring of blood gases is essential before weaning, which should not be considered until the following criteria are met:
   - Alveolar-arterial gradient of less than 300–350 mm Hg (40–45 kPa) while breathing 100% oxygen

- $PaCO_2 < 5.0$ kPa (a somewhat higher value, up to 6 kPa, may be accepted with chronic obstructed airway disease)
- V_D/V_T ratio < 0.6
- Arterial blood pH > 7.35
- $PaO_2 > 8$ kPa with $FIO_2 < 40\%$ and not more than 5 cm H_2O PEEP

2. Pulmonary function criteria:
   - On daily measurement *vital capacity* stable at 10 ml/kg, better 15 ml/kg body weight
   - Maximum inspiratory force greater than 20 cm H_2O
   - Consider IMV if tidal volume is below 7 ml/kg.
3. *Pulse oximetry* is a most valuable method of assessing the effectiveness of the patient's effort; saturation falling below 90% breathing air indicates support needed.
4. Stability of cardiovascular system
   Heart rate < 100/min in adults
5. Any increased oxygen consumption or carbon dioxide production associated with fever or shivering may make weaning impossible.
6. *State of consciousness* – the retention of consciousness and of an adequate cough and gag reflex is necessary before extubation.

When weaning starts the subject must be observed for at least 10 min; thereafter, half-hourly respiratory and circulatory parameters should be recorded.

Return to IPPV if:

- Heart rate or respiratory rate rise over the following 1.5 hours to > 120 and > 45 respectively.
- Hypoxia develops below 8 kPa or 91% saturation, or hypercarbia rises 1.5% above commencing level.
- Deteriorating level of consciousness is noted

Look for pyrexia and signs of bronchospasm and incipient pulmonary oedema.

E. Outline of Cardiopulmonary Resuscitation

1. Diagnose arrest by absent pulses, apnoea, or agonal gasping, dilating pupils.
2. A sharp precordial blow may restart asystolic heart or convert a ventricular tachy/bradycardia.
3. Give 400 watt/s direct countershock, if available.

4. Place board under patient's chest or move patient to the floor. As soon as possible, and as long as arrest persists:
   - Establish an airway; ventilate with oxygen 15–20 times/min; intubate trachea with cuffed tube as soon as feasible.
   - Closed chest massage applied 40–60 times/min synchronizing lung inflation with external chest compression; elevate legs; auscultate chest intermittently and if pneumothorax occurs, insert a tube thoracotomy; if closed chest massage is ineffective (trauma, deformity), open left chest through 5th intercostal space and initiate manual cardiac compression with one or both hands; all drugs except bicarbonate may be given directly into left ventricle (open chest).
   - Establish a large-bore i.v. and give 100 mEq $NaHCO_3$; give 50 mEq every 5 min or (better) as indicated by central venous or arterial blood-gas criteria.

The ABC of Resuscitation

A - Airway

B - Breathing

C - Cardiac massage

D - Diagnose
     Drugs*
     Defibrillation

E - Edema (cerebral)
     Electrolytes

* **A**drenaline **B**icarbonate **C**alcium Chloride **D**examethasone

---

5. Connect electrocardiograph; therapy pursued depends on rhythm obtained:
   - Asystole: give 1 mg adrenaline diluted in 10 ml saline intravenously, endotracheally (preferably), or intracardially. 1 g $CaCl_2$ (10 ml of 10%) intravenously: intracardiac injection is hazardous. Direct or intravenous pacemaker if available.
   - Ventricular tachycardia or fibrillation: administer direct current counter-shock 400 watt/s; lignocaine 50–100 mg intravenously or endotracheally if necessary.
   - Idioventricular rhythm: check pulse and blood pressure.
     - – Slow pulse: treat with 0.2 mg glycopyrrolate or 0.5 mg atropine (repeat as needed up to 4 ×); i.v. drip with isoproterenol or adrenaline. Check oxygen delivery.

- – Hypotension: use 10 ml of 10% $CaCl_2$ intravenously, or phenyl-ephrine, adrenaline, dopamine or dobutamine.
- Multifocal or unifocal ventricular extrasystoles: give 50–100 mg lignocaine intravenously.
- Supraventricular arrhythmia: check intravascular volume status; if digitalis intoxication (?) – give 100 mg diphenylhydantoin slowly intravenously.

6. Obtain a blood sample for:

A. Electrolytes; correct abnormalities.

B. Blood gases (arterial sample); correct hypoxia and hypercapnia; do not ventilate excessively ($PaCO_2$ less than 25 Torr).

III. Blood and Fluid Replacement

A. Normal Blood Volumes

Infant	90 ml/kg
Child	80 ml/kg
Adult female	60 ml/kg
Adult male	70 ml/kg

B. Significant Volume Losses

Compensation by capacitance vessels permits a variation in blood volume of $\pm 15\%$ in the normal individual without interstitial to vascular compartment fluid shift or other gross disturbance, but note that surgical patients may be volume depleted by starvation. With greater loss volume replacement takes priority over restoring red cell mass. RBC reserve is carried in blood. Tissue oxygen delivery is optimal at HCT of 30%, as the reduced viscosity lowers flow resistance. HCT should not fall below 25% or Hb < 7 g%

C. General Intravenous Fluid Requirements

These values provide rough guidelines. Trauma, nutritional state and disease states modify requirements, which should be checked by biochemical estimates.

(A) Water

1. Endogenous (metabolic) water	± 300 ml/24 h
2. Minimum obligatory urine volume	± 500 ml/24 h
3. Insensible evaporation loss from skin and respiratory tract – great variation with high ambient temperatures or pyrexia	± 500 ml/24 h

4. Fluid loss in stools	± 100 ml/24 h
5. Minimum daily water requirement	40 ml/kg/24 h
6. Water requirement during pre- and postoperative starvation	1.5–2.0 ml/kg/h
7. Paediatric requirements – up to	4.0 ml/kg/h

(B) Sodium

1. Minimum adult requirement	1.0–1.5 mEq/kg/24 h
or	70–100 mEq/24 h
going up to	200–300 mEq/24 h
depending on recent trauma, nutritional state	
2. Children:	2–3 mEq/kg/24 h

3. Sodium is lost particularly in secretions from gastrointestinal tract.
4. Diuretics increase renal losses.
5. Requirements of sodium, the extracellular cation, are reasonably accurately measured from serum electrolytes.

(C) Potassium

1. Minimum adult requirement 0.75–1.0 mEq/kg/24 h; this is influenced by carbohydrate metabolism.
2. Children: 2 mEq/kg/24 h
3. Potassium loss is greatly increased by many diuretics and by concomitant Mg deficiency.
4. Serum potassium levels are not good indicators of total body content.

(D) Magnesium

1. Normal daily requirement 0.3–0.35 mEq/kg/24 h. Magnesium is a positive inotropic agent.

(E) Calcium

Body stores are usually adequate for short-term requirements; otherwise, 0.22 mEq/kg/24 h.
Calcium requirements are influenced by phosphates.

(F) Phosphates

0.15–0.40 mEq/kg/24 h;
greatly influenced by nitrogen balance.

(G) Fuel Composition of 70-kg Man

(1 Kcal = 4.1868 kj)

Tissue stores	kg	kj
Fat (adipose triglyceride)	15	590000
Protein (mainly muscle)	6	100000
Glycogen (muscle)	0.150	2500
Glycogen (liver)	0.075	1250
		693750

Circulating fuels		
Glucose (in extracellular fluid)	0.020	335
Free fatty acids (plasma)	0.0003	13
Triglycerides (plasma)	0.003	126
		474

Normal daily energy requirement is 7500 kilojoule. During starvation at this rate of consumption circulatory fuels last about 6 h. Thereafter, tissue stores are mobilized:

Protein ± 6.4 g/h
Carbohydrate ± 2.6 g/h
Fat ± 5.6 g/h

D. Intraoperative Fluid Requirements

1. Use of vasodilators in premedication (droperidol or chlorpromazine) can unmask unexpected preoperative hypovolaemia and indicate need for preoperative fluid loading.
2. Infuse volume equivalent to 1.5–2.0 ml/kg/h for period of preoperative starvation before induction.
3. Maintain basic infusion rate 1.5 ml/kg/h during surgery.
4. Add to this:
   (a) Supplement for third space lesion – the extent depends on extent of surgical trauma, typically 1–2 litres for abdominal operations, developing during and within first 2–3 h after surgery.

   Recommended: 5–10 ml/kg/h up to 4 litres

   Severe rapid blood loss of >20% blood volume involves further depletion of extracellular fluid.

5. Use polyionic *resuscitation solutions* ("balanced salt solutions")
   Maintenance solutions are unsuitable for such fast infusion rates.
6. During major surgery monitor urine flow; infuse to maintain 1–2 ml/min excretion – maintain CVP 10–15 cm H_2O.
7. Infuse carbohydrate at 10 g/h (adult).
8. Suggested crystalloid administration (ml/kg/h of surgery)

Surgical trauma	Hour of surgery			
	1	2	3	4
Minimal (e.g. herniorraphy)	3– 5	2– 3	2–3	1–2
Moderate (e.g. gastric resection)	5– 8	4– 6	3–5	2–4
Severe (e.g. abdominal aneurysmectomy)	8–15	6–11	5–9	4–8

These provide only rough estimates of fluid requirement; they must be modified by additional data, e.g. urine output and osmolality, central venous pressure, and body temperature.
9. Blood loss is replaced in addition to this regime (see suggested treatment of blood loss during surgery, VII. H).

E. Neonatal and Paediatric Fluid Requirements*

During the first week of life, ECF space reduces from 36% to 25% of body mass. Daily fluid requirement stabilises only on 6th day.

Neonate requires:

1st to 5th day	50 ml/kg/24 h
6th day	150 ml/kg/24 h

Anaesthetic Routine

1. Correct starvation deficit: give 8 ml/kg in 5–20 min before induction.
2. Basic fluid requirement during surgery: 4 ml/kg/h
3. Third space lesion: totals 8–25 ml/kg given in addition during surgery.
4. All intraoperative fluids should contain 5% dextrose.
5. Correct meticulously for gastrointestinal fluid losses during surgery.

---

* By T.J.V. Voss

Postoperatively

0–10 kg	100 ml/kg/24 h
10–20 kg	1000 ml + 50 ml/kg/24 h
Above 20 kg	1500 ml + 20 ml/kg/24 h

Normal Birth Weight

1st day	30–60 ml/kg/24 h
2nd day	60
3rd day	90
4th day	90–150
1 year	120
1–2 years	100
2–4 years	85
4–10 years	70

Premature	*ml/kg/24 h*
1st day	60
2nd day	75
3rd day	90
4th day	105
5th day	120
6th day	135
7th day	150
8th day	165
9th day	195

Energy Requirements in Infancy and Childhood[1]

Age (years)	Energy needs	
	kJ/kg	kcal/g
0 –0.25	500	120
0.25–0.5	480	115
0.5 –1	460	110
1 –3	420	100
4 –6	380	90
7 –9	326	80
10–12 Boys	300	70
Girls	260	60
13–15 Boys	240	55
Girls	210	50

[1] Suggestions of the Food and Agricultural Organization of the World Health Organization

Body Fluid Compartments

	Neonate	Infant	Adult
Plasma	5%	5%	5%
Interstitial fluid	45%	30%	15%
Intracellular fluid	± 25%	40%	50%
Total body water	80%	75%	± 65%
Blood volume	85–100 ml/kg	80 ml/kg	70 ml/kg

Water turnover in infants is ± 15% of total body water per day.

Heat Loss and Thermoregulation

The environmental temperature at which body temperature can be maintained without protective clothing or the expenditure of extra energy is termed the "thermoneutral point". Infants rely on nonshivering thermogenesis in brown adipose tissue to generate heat – a sympathetic response.

Premature	34 °C
Neonate	32 °C
Infant	30 °C
Adult	28 °C

F. Standard Blood Orders for Elective Surgical Procedures

Major blood transfusion reactions arise from donor cell agglutination by recipient plasma. Present blood bank practice relies on Grouping and Screening techniques for preparing donor blood for transfusion. This involves:

1. Grouping of recipient blood for AB0 and Rh factors
2. Screening of recipient blood for red cell alloantibodies
3. Storage of recipient serum for possible later Crossmatching

Crossmatching does not materially add to safety of blood transfusion but increases costs.

Blood should thus be ordered after consideration of:

1. Expected blood loss with planned surgery
2. Patient's ability to handle blood loss (anaemia, low blood volume)
3. Unusual complicating factors

Four options may be exercised:
1. Book no blood
2. Group and screen
3. Crossmatch units against patient and each other
4. Retain serum for grouping and screening until after surgery

The following guidelines represent standard blood bank orders for common surgical procedures and are applicable for the majority of elective operations; the orders can be increased when increased blood needs are likely.

	None	G & S	Crossmatch (units)
Cardiothoracic surgery			
Arterial bypass procedures:			
– Aortofemoral and ileofemoral		×	
– Aortic (abdominal) aneurysm			4
– Femoral popliteal		×	
Bronchoscopy, mediastinoscopy	×		
Lobectomy, pneumectomy			2
Lung biopsy		×	
Pacemaker insertion	×		
Thoracotomy			2
Cardiopulmonary bypass		×	4
General Surgery			
Anal fissure, abscess (ischiorectal)	×		
Appendectomy	×		
Breast – biopsy, lumpectomy	×		
– mastectomy		×	
Cholecystectomy		×	
Colon/rectum resection		×	
Colostomy		×	
Common bile duct exploration		×	
Esophageal myotomy		×	
Gastrectomy, gastroplasty			2
Gastrostomy		×	
Haemorroidectomy	×		
Hernia repair (hiatus, incisional)		×	
Hernia repair (inguinal)	×		
Laparotomy		×	
Liver resection			6
Lumbar sympathectomy		×	
Lymph node biopsy	×		
Portocaval shunt			6
Splenectomy		×	

	None	G & S	Crossmatch (units)
Thyroidectomy, parathyroidectomy		×	
Vagotomy and pyloroplasty		×	
Whipple's procedure			6
Gynaecology			
Caesarean section		×	
Conization of cervix	×		
D & C	×		
Hysterectomy – vag. or abdominal		×	
Hysterectomy – Wertheim			6
Laparoscopy (colcoscopy)	×		
Oophorectomy		×	
Tubal ligation	×		
Vaginal repair/Marshall–Marchetti		×	
Neurosurgery			
Burr hole +/− needle biopsy		×	
Carotid endarterectomy		×	
Cranioplasty		×	
Craniotomy (tumour or aneurysm)			2
Discectomy		×	
ECIC bypass		×	
Hypophysectomy			2
Laminectomy (cervical or lumbar)		×	
Ventriculoperitoneal shunt		×	
Ophthalmology			
All procedures	×		
Otolaryngology			
Laryngoscopy	×		
Mastoidectomy	×		
Parotid tumour		×	
Tonsillectomy, adenoidectomy	×		
Orthopaedic surgery			
Amputation – below knee		×	
– above knee		×	
Arthroscopy	×		
Bone tumour resection			3
Discectomy		×	
Hip replacement (total)			3
Knee replacement (total)		×	
Laminectomy (cervical or lumbar)		×	
Meniscectomy	×		

	None	G & S	Crossmatch (units)
Patellectomy	×		
Putti-Platt procedure	×		
Scoliosis surgery			4
Spinal fusion			2
Plastic surgery			
Head or neck surgery		×	
Skin graft	×		
Skin or muscle flap			2
Urological surgery			
Bladder tumour – fulguration	×		
Cystectomy			4
Cystoscopy	×		
Ileal conduit		×	
Nephrectomy – simple		×	
Nephrolithotomy (anatrophic)			4
Orchidectomy	×		
Prostate needle biopsy	×		
Prostatectomy – transurethral		×	
– retropubic			2
Pyeloplasty		×	
Retroperitoneal lymph node dissection (radical)			4
Ureteral reimplantation		×	
Uterolithotomy	×		
Urethroplasty		×	
Vasectomy	×		
Medical Procedures			
Kidney biopsy		×	
Liver biopsy		×	

Note: G & S stands for "group and screen" and includes a blood group, antibody detection, and storage of serum for crossmatch.

One unit is approximately 400 ml whole blood.

This table is a modification of the recommendations drawn up by Dr. Robert Barr, Medical Director of the Canadian Red Cross, Blood Transfusion Service, London, Ontario Centre, and published as Kelten et al. [12].

G. Blood Products Available

1. Whole blood
   a. Fresh
   b. Standard – expiry 28 days
   c. Leucocyte poor
   d. Paediatric pack

2. Red cell concentrate (HCT = 70)
   a. Fresh
   b. Standard
   c. Washed
   d. Leucocyte poor
   e. Frozen
   f. Adsol. HCT 60% (mannitol, adenine, dextrose)

3. White cell concentrate

4. Plasma
   a. Dried
   b. Fresh frozen (all protein coagulation factors)
   c. Zoster immune
   d. Albumin 20%
   e. Immune serum globulin

5. Other products
   Cryoprecipitate
   Antihaemophilic factor
   Platelet concentrate

6. Fibrinogen

H. Suggested Treatment of Blood Loss During Surgery

Patients with a normal blood volume, a haemoglobin > 12 g/dl, and with measured loss not exceeding 15% of the blood volume will not require blood transfusion – only crystalloid transfusion. Since crystalloid is distributed throughout the extracellular fluid space and not confined to the vascular bed, replacement volume is approximately $3 \times$ loss.

Percentage of volume lost	Crystalloid		Blood
10	1– 3 times blood loss		Nil
10–20	1– 3 times blood loss	and	up to equiv. of red cell mass lost as packed cells
20–50	8–10 ml/kg/h	and	equiv. mass of red cells lost as packed cells. Reserve use of whole blood for special indications. Autotransfusion
50–100	8–10 ml/kg/h	and	equiv. volume of whole blood lost. Consider blood component usage and autotransfusion. Fresh-frozen plasma – 1 unit for each 4 blood units. Platelet count and transfusion if needed.

N. B.

1. Aim to keep haematocrit at 30% or higher.
2. Use 20–40 μm filters when 4 or more units of blood are to be transfused.
3. Losses of > 50% require additional clotting factors (FFP).
4. Colloid solutions alone should not be used for blood replacement (as opposed to volume replacement) because:
   a) Protein concentration of remaining blood is not significantly decreased
   b) Colloid does not replace extracellular fluid deficit that occurs with blood loss
   c) Expense
   d) May lead to late pulmonary problems
5. Optimal tissue oxygen delivery is achieved at a haematocrit of 30%, which so lowers the blood viscosity and therefore the peripheral resistance that a higher cardiac output is achieved without increased heart work.
6. Under steady state, volume to be transfused may be calculated:
   a) Based on haematocrit:
      - (Final HCT – measured HCT) $\times$ 2.5 $\times$ body wt. (kg) = ml whole blood
      - (Final HCT – measured HCT) $\times$ 1.5 $\times$ body wt. (kg) = ml packed cells
   b) Based on haemoglobin:
      - (Final Hb – measured Hb) $\times$ body wt. (kg) $\times$ 8 = ml whole blood
      - (Final Hb – measured Hb) $\times$ body wt. (kg) $\times$ 2 = ml packed cells

I. Composition of Representative Intravenous Solutions

Type	Cations				Anions					Substrate			pH	Osmol mosm/l	Free water
	Na⁺	K⁺	Mg⁺⁺	Ca⁺⁺	Cl	HPO₄	Lact	Acet	HCO₃	Gluconate	GM per litre	Kj			
Resuscitation															
Normal saline	154	–	–	–	154	–	–	–	–	–			5.5	308	–
Ringer's solution	147.5	4	–	4.5	156	–	–	–	–	–			6	309	–
Lactated Ringers soln	130	4	–	3	109	–	28	–	–	–		–	6.5	272	+
Plasmalyte A	140	5	3	–	98	–	–	27	–	23			7.4	294	–
Plasmalyte B	130	4	3	–	109	–	–	–	28	–		88	7.4	273	+
Plasmalyte R	140	10	3	–	98	–	–	27	–	23			7.4	294	–
Hidroliet	130	5.4	1.5	1.8	108	–	–	29	–	–	50	850	5	548	–
Normal Plasma	142	5	3	5	103	–	–	–	27	–			7.4	285	
Maintenance															
Darrow's solution	121	36	–	–	104	–	53	–	–	–	–	–	5	314	–
Normomfundin	100	18	6	4	90	–	–	38	–	–	50	850	5	536	–
Maintelyte	40	25	–	–	65	–	–	–	–	–	100	1700	4	684	–
Electrolyte No. 2	57	25	6	–	50	12.5	25	–	–	–	100	1700	5	723	–
Plasmalyte 56	40	13	3	–	40	–	–	16	–	–	–	–	5.5	110	+
Plasmalyte M	40	16	3	–	40	–	12	12	–	–	50	850	5.5	376	–
Neonatalyte	20	15	0.5	2.5	21	3.75	20	–	–	–	100	1700	4.2	670	–
Dextrose 10%	–	–	–	–	–	–	–	–	–	–	100	1700	5	560	+
Therapeutic															
Sodium bicarbonate 4.2%	500	–	–	–	–	–	–	–	500	–	–	–	7.9	1000	–
Sodium lactate inj. M/6	167	–	–	–	–	–	167	–	–	–	–	–	6.5	334	–
Hypertonic saline 5%	850	–	–	–	850	–	–	–	–	–	–	–		1700	–

94

Colloids	Cations				Anions						Substrate					
	Na+	K+	Mg++	Ca++	Cl	HPO4	Lact	Acet	HCO3	Gluconate	C.O.P. mm H2O	mol. wt.	pH	Osmol.	Half-life hours	Oncotic press mm H2O
LMW dextran 10% in saline	154	–	–	–	154	–	–	–	–	–		40000			1	
HMW dextran 6% + 5% dextrose	154	–	–	–	–	–	–	–	–	–		70000			12	
HMW dextran 6% in saline	154	–	–	–	154	–	–	–	–	–		70000			12	
Gelofusin	154	0.4	–	0.4	125	gelatin anion = 30 mEq/l										
Plasmagel 3% gelatin	142	–	2.8	–	80	–	gelatin anion = 64.8 mEq/l					35000	7.4		5	
Haemaccel 3.5% polygeline	145	5.1	–	12.5	145	+					350–390	35000	7.3	301	5	350–390
Hetastarch 6% in saline	154	–	–	–	154	–					435	450000	32 mmHg		>24	435
Human plasma fraction (4%)	150	2	near plasma concentrations of electrolytes				protein anion = 32 mEq/l				272		7.3	285	5–10 days	272
Albumin 5%	154				120						272	69000	7.2	285	5–10 days	
Stabilized human serum	120–140	3–4		1–1.5	120–140	Protein 5% – Albumin 3% + globulins								260	5–10 days	

Notes:

1 kilocalorie (Kcal) = 4.1868 kilojoules (Kj)

Various substrates may be added by manufacturer – dextrose, fructose, sorbitol, xylitol. These may increase osmolality, but being metabolized, present a water load rather than a fluid load to the kidney.

pH is adjusted by the manufacturer – all sugar containing solutions have an acidic pH to control caramelization during heat sterilization.

There is much conflicting information published on colloids and mean, maximum and minimum molecular weights vary with batch and manufacturer. Osmolality: the number of milliosmoles per kg water. Osmolarity: the number of milliosmoles per litre. Osmolarity varies with temperature of system, but Osmolality is independent of temperature, as is mass. Calculated Osmolarity: the sum of the osmotically active particles of solute per litre solvent. Colloid Osmotic Pressure (C.O.P.) Oncotic Pressure: the generally small osmotic effect of large solute molecules (protein, dextran and starch polymers) which do not readily diffuse through biological membranes.

J. Indications for Total Parenteral Nutrition

1. Nonfunctioning gastrointestinal tract (obstruction, surgery, fistula, infection)
2. Where patient's nutritional requirements are greater than can be taken by mouth (severe burns, multiple injuries, prolonged starvation)
3. Patient unable to accept oral or tube feeding (anorexia nervosa, confusional states, geriatrics)
4. Nutritional state of patient and duration of condition. A starvation period in excess of 72 h should not be permitted (5% dextrose solutions intravenously are starvation). Where a prolonged starvation period is anticipated, TPN should be commenced early.

K. Guidelines for Total Parenteral Nutrition (from Lee [13])

1. Daily requirement for a 70-kg patient is about 12560 kJ.
2. This requirement is provided equally by glucose and soybean oil emulsion:
   a) 50% Glucose 750 ml with insulin 120 U + KCl 80 mmol per 24 h (5.36 g/kg/day or 0.223 g/kg/h)
   b) 20% Intralipid 750 ml to provide 150 g fat (6280 kJ) (2.14 g/kg/day or 0.089 g/kg/h)
   c) Glucose administered as a 50-ml bolus each hour using central venous line
   d) At least 30% of energy requirement must be carbohydrate, and fat must not exceed 3–4 g/kg/day.
3. Minimum protein requirement 15 g nitrogen/day. Equivalent Travasol 8.5% 1000 ml.
   a) Postoperative period 0.22–0.24 g/kg/day yielding 188–197 kJ/kg/day
   b) After stress period 0.17 g/kg/day = 147 kJ/g/day.
   c) Overall energy/nitrogen ratio is optimally 837 kJ/g.
   d) Optimal nitrogen/potassium ratio = 1 g/5–6 mmol.
4. Fluid volume from above = 750 ml glucose
   750 ml Intralipid
   1000 ml Travasol 8.5%
5. Balance of fluid and electrolyte requirement supplied from Electrolyte No. 2 Solution to supply daily requirements Na^+, K^+, Mg^{2+}, Phosphate, Cl'.

6. Trace elements

Iron	0.5– 4 mg	Copper	0.5–2.0 mg
Zinc	5 – 7 mg	Manganese	1.5–3 mg
Iodine	100 –200 μg	Chromium	0.3–1 μg

7. Vitamins

Basic requirements per kg body weight per day

	Child	Adult
Thiamine	0.05 mg	0.02 mg
Riboflavine	0.1 mg	0.03 mg
Nicotinamide	1 mg	0.2 mg
Pyridoxine	0.1 mg	0.03 mg
Folic acid	20 μg	3 μg
Vitamin B_{12}	0.2 μg	0.03 μg
Pantothenic acid	1 mg	0.2 mg
Biotin	30 μg	0.5 μg
Vitamin C	3 mg	0.5 mg
Vitamin A	100 μg	10 μg
Vitamin D	2.5 μg	0.04 μg
Vitamin K	50 μg	2 μg
Vitamin E	1 IU	0.5 IU

The child requirements are for the second year of life and will decrease with age to the adult requirement at ± 15 years. Under stress conditions up to 10 times the above requirements may be needed.

L. Some Indications for Haemodynamic Monitoring and Manipulation

(A) Intra-arterial Blood Pressure

1. Cardiac and major vascular surgery
2. Lung surgery
3. Intracranial procedures
4. Major trauma
5. Hypotensive techniques
6. Patients with significant cardiac, pulmonary or metabolic lesions and obesity

(B) Central Venous Pressure

1. Expected large blood or extracellular fluid volume change
2. Potential preoperatively hypovolaemic patients
3. Trauma
4. Shock
5. Incipient or actual cardiac failure

A high internal jugular vein puncture site is preferable. Note the poor correlation between CVP and LAP in mitral valve disease ($r = 0.48$)

(C) Indications for Swann-Ganz Catheterization

The Swann-Ganz catheter provides a practical method of achieving optimal left ventricular filling pressures for optimal cardiac output, which is part of good intraoperative management in major surgery of all types.

1. Patient with
   a) moderate-severe CVS disease
   b) pulmonary disease
   c) major surgery
   Definitions of a, b and c:

   a) *CVS disease*
      - Ejection fraction 50%
      - LVEDP > 20 mmHg ⎫ Invasive
      - Angiographically confirmed coronary artery disease ⎭
      - Previous infarction with congestive cardiac failure
      - Rheumatic or congenital vascular disease ⎫ Clinical
      - Pulmonary hypertension or complicated systemic hypertension ⎭

   b) *Pulmonary disease*
      - FEV_1/FVC < 60% and abnormal blood gases
      - Abnormal lung functions in a patient who will be ventilated postoperatively

   c) *Major surgery*
      - Thoracotomy
      - Major vascular surgery
      - Major bowel resection
      - Major cancer surgery
      - Operations with potential for large blood or extracellular fluid volume change

2. Major surgery for geriatric patients (> 65 years) with ASA status $\geq$ II – intraoperative
   ASA status III – start preoperatively for optimal regulation of CVS function

3. Neurosurgery
   For diagnosis (acute rise in PAP) and treatment of air embolism
4. Intensive care unit
   a) Shock
   b) Myocardial infarction
   c) Liver failure
   d) Massive trauma
   e) Diffuse obstructive pulmonary disease with cor pulmonale

(D) Causes of Inaccurate Pulmonary Diastolic and Wedge Pressure Readings

1. Mitral valve stenosis interposes extra gradient to left ventricular filling pressure.
2. Pulmonary hypertension causes poor correlation with LA pressure.
3. Obstructive airway disease raises intrathoracic pressure.
4. IPPV and especially PEEP raise mean intrathoracic pressure.
5. Wedging catheter tip in zone 1 (West [35]) of lung.
6. Changing position of patient during series of measurements.

(E) Complications Associated with Haemodynamic Monitoring

1. Intra-arterial Lines
   a) Thin-walled Teflon cannulae can kink and obstruct.
   b) Thrombosis – 25% incidence if cannulae in position for less than 20 h; if longer, up to 50%
   c) Arterial dissection
   d) Trauma to nerves, veins, wrist
   e) Uncontrollable bleeding, ecchymosis
   f) Pain, arterial spasm
   g) Emboli, gangrene, necrosis
   h) Infection

Preference should be given to short 20-g Teflon cannulae. Use radial artery, provided Allen's test is satisfactory, or brachial artery.

2. Central Venous Lines
   a) Arterial puncture, haemorrhage
   b) Incorrect placement
   c) Haematoma
   d) Pneumothorax
   e) Infection, thrombus formation, embolism, SBE
   f) Damaged thoracic duct
   g) Various intracardiac complications
   h) Air embolism

3. Complications Associated with Premature Atrial Contraction (PAC)
   a) Ventricular extrasystole (17% malignant)
   b) Ventricular tachycardia, ventricular fibrillation
   c) Heart block
   d) Lung embolism or thrombus formation with infarction
   e) Pulmonary artery perforation, haemorrhage
   f) Rupture of balloon
   g) Damage to pulmonary valve, SBE
   h) Catheterization of carotid artery
   i) Knotting (do not insert more than 60 cm from IJV or 15 cm past RV)
   j) Right heart valve vegetations may be dislodged or block passage of catheter
   k) Infection – systemic and local

(E) Cardiovascular Manipulations

Using the monitoring lines available, one may diagnose one of the three main haemodynamic problems: hypovolaemia, fluid overload, or cardiac failure, by the use of an intravenous fluid challenge.

1. Using Central Venous Pressure Monitoring

CVP reading (cm H_2O)	i.v. Fluid load over 10 min
< 8	200 ml
8–12	100 ml
> 12	50 ml

Response pattern may be a pressure rise of (cm H_2O)
a) < 3 : repeat
b) 3–5 : wait and reassess
c) > 5 : stop test

2. Using Pulmonary Artery Pressure Monitoring (mm Hg)

PAWP (mm Hg)	i.v. Fluid load
< 12	200 ml
12–16	100 ml
> 16	50 ml

Response pattern may be a pressure rise of (mm Hg)
a) < 5 : repeat
b) 5–7 : wait and reassess
c) > 7 : stop test
Response **a** indicates hypovolaemia with good handling of fluid load.

Response **b** correlated with the fluid load may indicate either adequate hydration (200 ml) or inability of the heart to handle a fluid load (50 ml).

Response **c** after any one of the three fluid loads, but especially with raised CVP or PAC pressures, indicates a failing heart.

3. Treatment Indicated by Derived Parameters

↑	Stable	Circulatory overload?
	No treatment	Diuretics
LVSWI $(gm\,m/m^2)\,20$ or $2,5\ l/m^2/min$ CI		Venodilatation (↓ preload)
	Hypovolaemia	Failing Heart?
	Fluid challenge	Reduce preload
		Reduce afterload
		Inotropic support

↑ 0   or   ⟶ 18 mm Hg ⟶
PAWP

Chapter 3

I. Drugs and Doses

A. Standard Drugs and Doses in Anaesthesia

1. General Inhalation Agents

The dose of inhalational agents does not vary with the weight of the patient as is the case with parenteral and oral drugs. Gases dissolve according to a constant solubility coefficient in plasma which varies little with age or mass. Factors that potentiate inhalational drugs include:

a) Age – particularly advanced
b) Shock – distribution of the drug throughout the body is preferential to the central nervous system and other essential organs; body cells in general are more sensitive as a result of hypoxia.
c) Damage to or overstress of organ systems increases sensitivity – particularly significant in circulatory and respiratory systems
d) Previous drug therapy – sedatives, neuroleptics, narcotics, antihypertensives, beta blockers

The dose of inhalational agents is based on two systems:

– **MAC** – Mean alveolar concentration is that concentration that will keep 50% of patients asleep and non-reactive to surgical stimulus after complete equilibration. This is also called the AD50 – Anaesthetic Dose 50%.
– **AD95** – The concentration of the drug which after complete equilibration, will keep 95% of patients still during surgery. This is a far more practical figure. (Note that oxygen is here the carrying gas.)

	AD50	AD95
Ether	1.92	2.22
Cyclopropane (sea level)	9.14	10.1
Halothane	0.74	0.90
Methoxyflurane (Penthrane)	0.16	0.22
Fluroxene (Fluoromar)	3.40	3.57
Enflurane (Ethrane)	1.69	1.88
Isoflurane (Forane)	1.16	1.63

The practical significance of these figures:

a) AD50 is a suitable concentration with a nitrous oxide/oxygen mixture of 60/40.

b) AD95 is a suitable concentration with pure oxygen as a carrying gas.

Both figures apply only after complete body saturation after induction, and they are also influenced by premedication.

2. Paediatric Considerations

Drug doses given to children are based upon (a) body weight (usually), or (b) surface area, which is preferable in small children. The unit is m^2. Age is an *unreliable* guide to dosage.

Dosage is more commonly based on the adult dose assuming adult BSA = 2 m^2 or adult weight is 70 kg. For healthy young children one can assume that:

– at 1 year the child is $\frac{1}{10}$ adult weight
– at 2 years the child is $\frac{2}{10}$ adult weight
– at 3 years the child is $\frac{2.5}{10}$ adult weight
– at 6 years the child is $\frac{3}{10}$ adult weight

DuBois' formula

BSA (D) = $h^{0.725}$ (cm) × $W^{0.425}$ (kg) 71.84 × 10^{-4} (m^2)

Boyde's formula (The DuBois formula will produce large error for a child when BSA is smaller than 0.6 m^2.)

BSA = $h^{0.3}$ (cm) × $W^{(0.7285 - 0.0188 \log w)}$ (g) × 3.207 × 10^{-4} (m^2)

Normal 95th percentile growth rates are (in kilograms):

	Male	Female		Male	Female		Male	Female
1 month	5	4	2 years	12.5	12	10 years	33	33
3 months	6	5.5	4 years	17	16	12 years	40	42
6 months	8	7.5	6 years	21	10	14 years	50	50
1 year	10	9.5	8 years	25	25	18 years	70	57

3. General Intravenous Induction Agents

Agent	mg/kg i.v.	Average mg for a 70-kg person
Thiopentone	4–5	250
Methohexitone	1–1.5	100
Propofol	2.5	175
Etomidate	0.2–0.3	10–20

Agent	mg/kg i. v.	Average mg for a 70-kg person
Gamma-OH (gamma-hydroxybutyric acid)	50	3000
Ketamine	2–3	150 (effective as i. m. injection 5–10 mg/kg)
Morphine	1–3	70–200 ⎫ in these doses
Fentanyl	10–50 μg	1 ⎪ always apnoea
Sufentanil	8–30 μg	1 ⎬ and often
Alfentanil	40–100 μg	4 ⎭ muscle rigidity
Diazepam	0.25–0.5 mg	20
Lorazepam	0.6 mg	4
Midazolam	0.15–0.3 mg	10–15

Several of these drugs are used in other applications at lower doses. Dose will vary according to physical status and age.

Specific antagonists are available for the opiate group – naloxone and naltrexone – and will become available for the benzodiazepine group. Physostigmine, having a central cholinergic action, has been used in the reversal of ketamine, hyoscine and benzodiazepines, but lacks specificity.

4. Muscle Relaxants

a. Depolarising drugs

Suxamethonium Cl (Scoline)	1–1.5	70–100
Suxamethonium Br (Brevidil M)	1–1.5	60 cation
Suxethonium Cl (Brevidil E)	1.5–1.75	100 cation

b. Nondepolarising drugs

	Precurarising test dose	90% relaxation	mg/70 kg
Gallamine (Flaxedil)	20–30 mg (adult dose)	1.5–2 mg/kg	120–160
Alcuronium (Alloferin)	2.5 mg (adult dose)	0.25 mg/kg	15–20
Pancuronium (Pavulon)	0.5 mg (adult dose)	0.08–0.1 mg/kg	6–8
Dextro-Tubocurarine (Tubarine)	5–7 mg (adult dose)	0.5 mg/kg	30–40
Atracurium (Tracrium)		0.5–0.6 mg/kg ⎫	
Vecuronium (Vecuron)		0.08–0.1 mg/kg ⎬ equipotent doses	
Metocurine		0.3–0.4 mg/kg ⎭	

Follow-up doses of nondepolarisers: ⅓ of the original full curarising dose except in the case of Pavulon, where ⅛–⅒ of the original dose is sufficient.

The precurarising dose of one of the above agents is sometimes given before suxamethonium to reduce fasciculations, muscle pain, and bradycardia.

c. Direct-acting muscle relaxants

Dantrolene   2.5 mg/kg
(Used as treatment for malignant hypothermia)

d. Antidotes for nondepolarisers

These are short- to medium-acting cholinesterases.

	mg/kg	mg/70 kg
Edrophonium (Tensilon) test dose	0.12–0.16	10–15
Edrophonium full-reversal dose	0.5–1.5	30–100
Neostigmine (Prostigmine)	0.03–0.06	2.5–5
Pyridostigmine (Mestinon)	0.06–0.12	5–10

Antimuscarinic drugs must always be given with these dose scales, except for the edrophonium (Tensilon) test dose.

Atropine with anticholinesterase:	0.02–0.03	1.5–2
Glycopyrrolate (Robinul)	0.005–0.01	0.4–0.8
	or 0.2 mg with	
	each 1 mg	
	neostigmine	

5. Local Analgesic Drugs

a) The concentration of the drug must be suitable to block the desired nerve. A thicker nerve requires a greater concentration in solution. In the case of lignocaine:

Subcutaneous	0.25%
Small nerve	0.5%
Ulnar nerve	1.0%
Epidural	1.5%
Brachial plexus	2.0%
Spinal block	5.0%

b) The total dose administered must be strictly limited to avoid toxic effects. Toxicity is influenced by:
   – Richness of the blood supply in the area involved (NB: The head and neck have an extremely rich blood supply; thus, infiltrations in this area have a higher toxicity.)

- Concentration – with a higher concentration there is a higher gradient to the bloodstream from the area where the drug is deposited, and this will accelerate uptake and increase toxicity.
- Adrenaline is given for vasoconstriction; it will delay absorption, and reduce toxicity.
- Protein binding – this is particularly significant in the case of bupivacaine, which has its toxicity thus reduced.
- Length of time between injections, and thus rate of degradation of drug

c) *Maximum Safe Doses for Commonly Used Infiltration Drugs*

Drug	Concentration (%)	Plain (mg/kg)	+ Adrenaline (mg/kg)	Max. dose per 70 kg with adrenaline (mg)	Max. in 24 h (mg)
Procaine	0.5–2	7	10	700	*
Chloroprocaine	0.5–2	11	14	1000	*
Lignocaine	0.5–2	4.5	7	500	half-life 1.5 h
Prilocaine	0.5–3	6	9	600	–
Mepivacaine	0.5–2	5.5	NA	500	1000
Bupivacaine	0.25–0.5	2.5	3.5	250	400

* A "procaine unit" – 4 mg/kg – can be given every 20 min. Chloroprocaine is four times as rapidly metabolized as procaine.

Prilocaine may cause methaemoglobinaemia at maximum dose.

d) *Regional Anaesthesia for Surgery of Limbs Under Tourniquent*
   Arm: 1–2 mg/kg of a 0.25% solution lignocaine
   Leg: 3–4 mg/kg of a 0.25% solution lignocaine

6. Premedicants

A large variety of drugs is used for this purpose including:
- Tranquillizers
- Antiemetics
- Opiates
- Atropine-like drugs
- Antihistamines

It is a good rule to reduce the dose of individual drugs when used together in a mixture.

Opiates are usually given in smaller than normal doses before operation, particularly where it is required that a patient should breathe spontaneously while under anaesthesia.

a) Phenothiazines

In various combinations these drugs offer antiemetic, antihistamine, antiadrenergic, sedative and atropine-like effects. Some potentiate opiate analgesia; others may be mildly antanalgesic but may not be significant once anaesthesia is established.

	i.m. dose (mg/kg)	70-kg dose (mg)
Promethazine (Phenergan)	0.4–0.6 mg/kg	25–50 mg
Chlorpromazine (Largactil)	0.2–0.4 mg/kg	12.5–25 mg
Trifluoperazine (Stelazine)	0.015 mg/kg	1–2 mg
Promazine (Sparine)	0.4–0.6 mg/kg	25–50 mg
Trimeprazine (Vallergan)	per os 2 mg/kg	only children
Droperidol (Inapsin)	0.15 mg/kg	10 mg
Hydroxyzine (Aterax)	0.7–1.5	50–100

b) Benzodiazepines:

	per os (mg/kg)	dosage mg/kg 70 kg	i.m.	remarks
Half-life <6 h				
Midazolam (Dormicum)	0.1–0.15	1–10	X	
Triazolam (Halcion)	1–15 µg	0.25–0.5		
Half-life 6–12 h				
Lormetazepam (Noctamid)	15 µg	1.0		
Loprazolam (Dormonoct)	15–30 µg	1–2		
Oxazepam (Serepax)	0.15–0.3	10–20		
Temazepam (Normison, Euhypnos)	0.2–0.4	15–30		
Half-life 12–24 h				
Alprazolam (Xanor)	4–8 µg	0.25–0.5		
Bromazepam (Lexotan)	30–80 µg	2–6		
Lorazepam (Ativan)	15–40 µg	1.0–2.5	X	
Half-life >24 h				
Chlordiazepoxide (Librium)	1.0–1.5	75–100		AM
Clobazam (Urbanol)	0.15	10		AM
Clonazam (Rivotril)	7–30 µg	0.5–2.0		Anticonvulsant
Clorazepate (Tranxene)	0.2–0.5	15–30		AM
Diazepam (Valium)	0.15–0.2	10–15	X	AM

	per os (mg/kg)	dosage mg/kg 70 kg	i.m.	remarks
Flunitrazepam (Rohypnol)	0.015–0.03	1–2	X	AM
Flurazepam (Dalmadorm)	0.2–1.0	15–60		AM
Ketazolam (Solatran)	0.2–0.5	15–30		
Medazepam (Nobrium)	0.1–0.15	5–10		AM
Nitrazepam (Mogadon)	0.1–0.15	5–10		
Prazepam (Demetrin)	0.15	10		AM

AM = This drug is biotransformed to an active metabolite.

Note: This is an extensive list of drugs in this category. For premedication shorter-acting drugs are preferred to reduce postoperative interaction with analgesics, opiates and sedatives. Some benzodiazepines may enhance opiate respiratory depression. For a good review see Van Rooyen and Offermeier [34].

c) Opiates

	Premedication (mg/kg)	Postoperatively (mg/kg)
Pethidine	0.5	1.0
Morphine	0.15	0.3
Papaveretum (Omnopon)	0.3	0.4
Oxymorphone (Numorphan)	0.01	0.02
Fentanyl (Sublimaze)	0.0015	0.003
Methadone (Physeptone)	0.15	0.2
MST continuous (Morphine)	10-mg and 30-mg tablets only for oral use – about 12 h action	

Agonists/antagonists as premedicants produce less respiratory depression but may interfere with i.v. opiates given as analgesic supplements.

Tilidine (oral – children)	0.5	1.0
Buprenorphine	0.0085	0.001
Nalbuphine	0.3	0.6
Ketamine	as postoperative analgesia	0.25

d) Atropine-like Drugs

Atropine	0.02–0.04	0.5–1.0
Scopolamine	0.05–0.08	0.4–0.6
Atropine per os	0.7–0.15	
Glycopyrrolate	0.003–0.005	0.2

7. Antiemetics

1. Antidopaminergic drugs acting purely on chemoreceptor trigger zone and gastric emptying:

Metoclopramide	0.15–0.5 mg/kg
Domperidone	0.15–1.0 mg/kg
Chlorpromazine	0.15–0.5 mg/kg

2. Anticholinergic drugs active in motion sickness:

Chlorpromazine	(mixed action)
Perphenazine	0.05–0.1 mg/kg
Prochlorperazine	0.1–0.2 mg/kg
Cyclizine	0.5–1.0 mg/kg
Dimenhydrinate	0.5–1.0 mg/kg

3. Anti-H_2 receptors for reduction of acid gastric secretion:

Cimetidine	1000–2000 mg/daily
Glycopyrrolate	0.005–0.1 mg/kg
Ranitidine	150 mg 12-hourly

8. Vasopressors

Vasopressors may have a pure alpha (noradrenaline) or pure beta (isoprenaline) or a mixed alpha and beta effect. Only pure alpha adrenergic drugs are safe with halothane, cyclopropane, etc., but excessive doses always produce both alpha and beta effects with all drugs. Any beta agonist given in high enough dose will produce alpha stimulation.

	i.v.	i.m.	Duration i.v. effect/min
Methoxamine (Vasoxine) $\alpha + \beta -$	5	20	15
Phenylephrine $\alpha + \beta 0$	0.5–1.0	5–10	10
Mephentermine (Wyamine) $\alpha + \beta +$	3	25	10
Metaraminol (Aramine) $\alpha + \beta +$	0.5–1.0	5–10	10
Ephedrine $\alpha + \beta +$	15–20	30–60	30–45
Etilefrine (Effortil) $\alpha + \beta +$	1–5	10	±20
Isoprenaline (Isuprel) $\alpha 0 \beta +$	0.4 mg dissolved in 200 ml Ringers and administered i.v. with a mini dripper gives optimal effect with control of tachycardia (one ampoule is equivalent to 0.2 mg)		
Dopamine (Intropin) $\alpha 0 \beta +$	250 mg dissolved in 200 ml, as above		
Dobutamine (Dobutrex) $\alpha 0 \beta +$	250 mg dissolved in 200 ml, as above		
POR-8 (Vasopressin)	Is not a catecholamine but an octapeptide and is used exclusively for tissue infiltration – 5 IU (1 ampoule) in not less than 30 ml Ringers solution.		

	i.v.	i.m.	Duration i.v. effect/min
Inocor (Amrinone)	i.v. Bolus of 0.5–1.5 mg/kg or as infusion of i.v. 100 mg dissolved in 200 ml Ringers/dextrose + H_2O. Titrate for desired effect. Has apparent beta action		

+, agonist; −, antagonist; 0, no effect

B. Opioid Receptors and Agonists

Receptor pure agonist	Effects	Available agonists and brain areas
Mu receptor	Dominant central depressive effects:	Morphine
	– Supraspinal analgesia (µl only)	Buprenorphine
	– Respiratory depression	Nalbuphine
Beta-Endorphin	– Hypothermia and bradycardia	
	– Euphoria and physical dependence	cerebral cortex hypothalamus, brain stem and spinal cord
(Met)enkephalin	– Miosis and catalepsy	
	– Increased locomotion	
	– Testosterone and LH inhibition	
	Peripheral effects:	
	– Decreased GI motility	
	– Baroceptor inhibition	
Kappa receptor	Sedative effects:	Ethylketazocine
	– Spinal analgesia	Nalbuphine
	– Dysphoria and sedation	Butorfanol
Dynorphin	– No respiratory depression	Pentazocine
	– Miosis	
	– Decreased motor activity	
	– ADH inhibition	hypothalamus, thalamus and spinal cord
	– Spinal injury and haemorrhagic shock	
	– Appetite suppression	
Sigma receptor	Dominant central stimulation:	Phencyclidine
	– Tachycardia and tachypnoea	Nalorphine
May not be exclusively opioid	– Dysphoria and hallucinations	Cyclazocine
	– Mydriasis and nausea	
	– No analgesia	corpus striatum brain stem and spinal cord
	– Increased motor activity	

Receptor pure agonist	Effects	Available agonists and brain areas
Delta receptor	– Spinal analgesia	
	– Stress-induced analgesia	
	– Growth hormone release	
(Leu)enkephalin	– Respiratory depression	
	– Hyperthermia	
	– Endotoxic and haemorrhagic shock	
	– LH and testosterone inhibition	
	– Hypotension	

The development of tolerance is a feature of all receptors. All have anticonvulsant effects.

Naloxone is a selective antagonist at all sites in decreasing order of potency mu → delta → kappa but not sigma. Nalorphine is a mu antagonist only.

C. Total Intravenous Anaesthesia

Indications

1. Prevention of atmospheric pollution in operating theatres
2. Where high FIO_2, mixtures are especially indicated
3. When it is undesirable to block the hypoxic vasoconstrictor reflex with volatile agents
4. In the absence of conventional anaesthetic equipment
5. For emergency surgery in confined areas or where explosion hazard exists

Techniques

Ideal technique relies on the use of noncumulative drugs. As there are currently no satisfactory monoanaesthetics, practical methods use monoaction drugs in combination – sleep, analgesia, relaxation, as in T.C. Gray's concept of balanced anaesthesia [9]. Oxygen-enriched air is the breathed gas mixture.

1. Propofol/Opiate

Propofol (Diprivan) is currently the intravenous anaesthetic with the shortest halflife in the body, lending itself to total intravenous anaesthetic (TIVA) techniques.

Premedication: Benzodiazepine and/or opiate.

Simple Procedures with Spontaneous Respiration:
a) Induction: Propofol 2.0–2.5 mg/kg bolus
b) Maintenance: Propofol infusion 9 mg/kg/h for 30 minutes
       thereafter 6 mg/kg/h
       with nitrous oxide and oxygen

Standard TIVA Technique:
a) Induction: Propofol 1.0–2.5 mg/kg
       Alfentanil 20 µg/kg (up to 100 µg/kg)
       Relaxant of choice and intubation
b) Maintenance: Propofol infusion 0.15 mg/kg/min (9 mg/kg/h)
       Alfentanil infusion 1 µg/kg/min (60 µg/kg/h)
       Ventilation with oxygen enriched air.

The infusions can be stopped 10–15 minutes before the end of surgery. With such dose schedules only reversal of relaxation but not of the opiate is indicated.

Standard Sedation During Regional Analgesia:
Propofol 6 mg/kg/h with spontaneous respiration.

2. Midazolam/Ketamine

Ketamine is used here as an analgesic in subanaesthetic doses. Although hallucinogenic effects should not be reached at the suggested doses, the concommitant use of midazolam is valuable for its amnesic and anti-hallucinogenic properties.

a) Premedication: to include Midazolam 0.1 mg/kg
       Glycopyrrolate 0.003 mg/kg
b) Induction: Midazolam 0.15 mg/kg
       Ketamine 1.0–1.5 mg/kg
c) Maintenance: Midazolam 0.05–0.1 mg/kg/h
       Ketamine 0.5–1.0 mg/kg/h

Note: Both Ketamine and midazolam are relatively long acting drugs, so postoperative recovery is slow. The use of reduced doses with nitrous oxide/oxygen may thus be desirable.

Ketamine levels show a biphasic decline with an initial fast phase of half-life 11 minutes and a slow phase of 2.5 hours.

Midazolam has an elimination halflife of ±2.5 hours (up to 5 hours in the elderly).

Dose rates will be considerably influenced by premedication, e.g. opiates *and in particular by droperidol.*

3. Ketamine/Nitrous Oxide

a) Premedication to include benzodiazepine, atropine, opiate
b) Induction with 1–2 mg/kg ketamine and nitrous oxide 75%
c) Maintenance: *System 1:*
  - use i.v. infusion of 1 mg/ml ketamine concentration
  - set drip rate (20 dr/ml) to the weight in kg
  - inhalation of 50% nitrous oxide in oxygen
  - for postoperative analgesia set rate to kg/10

  System 2:
  - use i.v. infusion concentration of $5 \times$ kg in 200 ml
  - drip rate of 60 dr/ml set – dose in μg/kg/min
  - inhalation of 50% nitrous oxide in oxygen
  - maintenance 5–15 μg/kg/min with nitrous oxide
  - normal maintenance dose 25–40 μg/kg/min with oxygen

4. Etomidate/Opiate

Etomidate approaches the ideal for this technique in that it is rapidly metabolized and noncumulative, does not release histamine, and produces relatively few undesirable side effects. It has *NO* analgesic properties.

Note: The use of etomidate infusions has been criticized because of the adrenal cortical suppression the drug produces. This side effect may be prevented by IV ascorbic acid [1a].

a) Premedication: To include opiate unless intravenous bolus is given prior to induction. Droperidol considerably potentiates etomidate.

b) Induction: Etomidate 0.1–0.3 mg/kg (greatly influenced by premedication). Alternatively an infusion of etomidate 100–150 μg/kg/min is given for 10 min followed by 10–15 μg/kg/min for maintenance.
  Opiate-fentanyl 0.1–0.2 μg/kg or Alfentanil 0.5–1.0 μg/kg
  Relaxant: as required
  With controlled ventilation higher opiate concentrations are given – fentanyl 10 μg/kg and Alfentanil 50 μg/kg after which spontaneous breathing returns in less than 60 min.

c) Maintenance: Etomidate 10–20 μg/kg/min
  Fentanyl 0.05–0.06 μg/kg/min (cumulative over several hours)
  Alfentanil 0.1 μg/kg/min (1 mg every 20 min)

It is important to state that there are no well-defined guidelines for total intravenous anaesthesia as there are with inhalation techniques, for the very good reason that blood levels of intravenously administered drugs are never as predictable as with inhalation drugs where an equilibrium across the alveolar membrane can be established. With a TIVA technique that includes muscle relaxants, awareness during anaesthesia is a possibility never to be disregarded [29].

D. Action of Antiarrhythmic Drugs

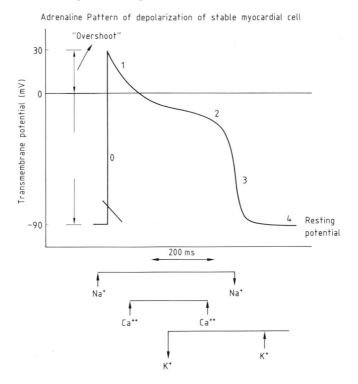

Adrenaline Pattern of depolarization of stable myocardial cell

Action potential of pacemaker cell showing spontaneous depolarization

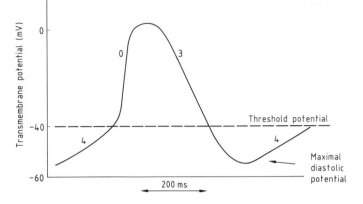

The influence of acetylcholine on pacemaker cells

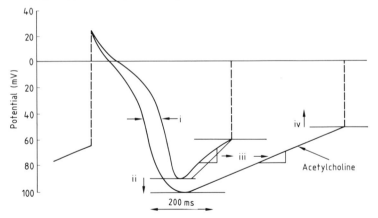

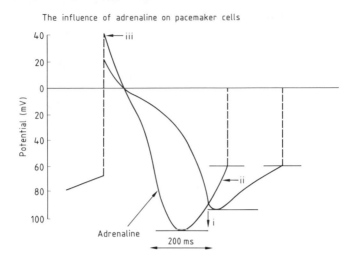

The influence of adrenaline on pacemaker cells

Potential (mV)

Adrenaline

200 ms

E. Antiarrhythmic Drugs

Classification:

Class I Membrane stabilising drugs

(A) Action: Probable decrease in membrane permeability for Na^+

1. Quinidine orally 15–30 g/kg/day in divided doses
2. Procainamide (Pronestyl) 1.5 mg/kg i.v. over 2 min followed by 0.3 mg/kg/min
3. Disopyramide (Rhythmodan) 2 mg/kg i.v. over 5 min to maximum of 150 mg

(B) Action: Probable decrease in membrane permeability for K^+

1. Diphenylhydantoin (Epanutin) 50–100 mg i.v. slowly every 5 min to maximum of 1 g
2. Lignocaine (Xylocaine) 1.5 mg/kg as bolus dose i.v.
   120 µg/kg/min as rapid infusion for 25 min
   30 µg/kg/min as maintenance infusion
   In congestive heart failure dosage must be reduced by 25%–50%.
3. Mexiletine (Mexitil) 150–250 mg over 5 min
   Not more than 750 mg over 3 h

Class II β-Blocking agents
> Action: Prolonging spontaneous depolarisation

(A) Cardioselective (β1)
1. Practolol (Eraldin) (i.v. use only) 30–100 μg/kg titrated
2. Atenolol (Tenormin) 100 mg orally daily
3. Acebutolol (Sectral) 12.5–50 mg i.v.

These drugs are preferred when bronchospasm is possible.

(B) Noncardioselective
1. Propranolol (Inderal) 1–10 mg i.v.
2. Sotalol (Sotacor) 10–20 mg i.v.
3. Pindolol (Visken) 0.4–2 mg i.v.
4. Oxprenalol (Trasicor) 1–12 mg i.v. } Titrate
5. Timolol (Blocadren) 0.4–1 mg i.v.
6. Alprenol (Aptin) 5–20 mg i.v.

Labetolol (Trandate) – noncardioselective with α blocking activity.
β to α-adrenergic blocking activity:
Per os 3:1   Intravenous 7:1
Main anaesthetic use: to control blood pressure without tachycardia

Class III Drugs that prolong action potential as their major effect
1. Amiodarone (Cordarone) 300–600 mg/day orally
2. Bretylium tosylate (Darenthin) i.v. or i.m. 5–10 mg/kg; repeat to maximum of 30 mg/kg

Class IV Calcium antagonists
> Action: Decrease plateau phase of action potential by inhibiting calcium transport over the membrane

1. Verapamil (Isoptin)   80–160 mg p.o.
                              75–200 μg/kg i.v.
2. Diltiazem (Tilazem)   60–120 mg p.o.
                              75–150 μg/kg i.v.
3. Nifedipine (Adalat)   10–30 mg p.o.
                              3–15 μg/kg i.v.

Class V Cardiac glycosides
> Action: Inhibit Na^+ and K^+-ATP-ase enzyme system. In increasing doses they first have a vagotonic effect, then an antisympathomimetic effect, and eventually direct suppression of SA and AV node.

1. Digoxin: Loading dose i.v. is 0.75–1 mg
   Oral loading dose 1 mg; not always necessary
   Maintenance dose 0.125–0.25 mg daily
2. Digitoxin: Start and maintain patient on 0.1–0.15 mg daily

120

Class VI Bradycardia relieving agents
Action: Acetylcholine blockade or β adrenergic agonist action shortening spontaneous depolarisation

1. Atropine 0.02-0.03 mg/kg
2. Glycopyrrolate 0.005-0.01 mg/kg
3. Inotropic drugs
4. Phosphodiesterase inhibition

Contraindications to beta-blockers
1. Left ventricular failure
2. Heart block
3. Bronchospasm in asthmatic patients
4. Gangrene
5. Liver diseases (avoid agents with high hepatic clearance)
6. Diabetes mellitus
7. Avoid propranolol in severe depression

F. Vasodilators

	i.v. dose	Duration
1. α Blockers		
a) Phentolamine (Regitine)	5-10 mg	10 min
b) Phenoxybenzamine (Dibenzyline)	0.5-2.0 mg/kg	24 h
c) Prazosin (Minipress)	0.5-2.0 mg orally	
d) Labetolol (Trandate)	1-2 mg/kg	±6 h
e) Chlorpromazine (Largactil)	2.5 mg increments	±6 h
2. Ganglion blocking agents		
a) Trimetaphan (Arfonad)	200 mg in 200 ml – given as slow i.v. infusion Stat. dose: 0.3-0.7 mg/kg i.v. (20-50 mg)	
b) Pentolinium (Ansolysen)	3-20 mg stat. i.v. titrated	
c) Guanethidine (Ismelin)	10-20 mg slowly i.m. or i.v.	

	i.v. dose	Duration

3. Smooth-muscle relaxants

a) Nitrates
- Nitroglycerin — 0.6-10 mg/h in solution
- Amyl nitrate (as inhalation) — 2-5 mg — 10 min
- Isosorbide dinitrate (Isordil) — 1-4 mg/h

b) Nitroprusside sodium — 20 mg nitroprusside in 200 ml 5% dextrose and water. Protect against light. Prepare fresh solution after 4 h. Start with 0.5 µg/kg/min. Increase gradually to 40-60 µg/kg/min. Titrate against blood pressure. Use practolol or labetolol to control tachycardia and rebound hypertension.

c) Hydralazine — 5-7.5 mg bolus

4. β-Stimulants

a) Isoprenaline (Isuprel) — 0.4 mg in 200 ml dextrose and water intravenously

b) Dobutamine (Dobutrex) ⎫
c) Dopamine (Intropin) ⎬ 250 mg in 200 ml as above
d) Salbutamol (Ventolin) — 0.1-0.4 µg/kg/min

Note: Dopamine preferred for renal vasodilation
Dobutamine produces less tachycardia

5. Angiotensin II inhibitors

Captopril (Capoten) — Available as tablets
No fixed guidelines
Up to 2 mg/kg/day

6. Central stimulants with peripheral actions

a) Methyldopa (Aldomet) — 50 mg slowly i.v.
b) Clonidine (Catapress) — Available as tablets

7. Calcium antagonists
See under "Antiarrhythmic Drugs"

Vasodilator drugs are titrated according to the response of a patient's blood pressure. They may be used in combination with β-blocking drugs to prevent compensatory tachycardia and renin release.

G. Some Preferred Drugs for Caesarean Section

1. Antacid   *Hydrotalcite (Altacite)*
2 g 0.5–2 h preoperatively
Maintains *neutral* gastric pH
Adsorbs bile, trypsin

2. Antisialogogue   *Glycopyrrolate (Robinul)*
0.2 mg 0.5–1.5 h preoperatively
Antisialogogue is better, less tachycardia
than atropine
Does not cross placenta
Reduces gastric acid secretion, but reduces lower oesophageal sphincter tone

3. Antiemetic   *Domperidone*
0.5 mg/kg
Increases lower oesophageal sphincter
tone and rate of gastric emptying
No extrapyramidal symptoms
Does not cross blood-brain barrier

4. Gastric-Acid Suppression   *Rantidine Zantac*

5. Induction Agent   *Ketamine*
1.5 mg/kg
Single dose for induction only
Longest period of amnesia in mother
with least effect on infant
Raises BP, thus contraindicated in pre-
eclampsia or with extreme tachycardia
Thiopentone alternative; 4 mg/kg single
induction dose

6. Inhalation Agents   Oxygen 50% minimum concentration in
nitrous oxide. Enflurane 0.5–1.0% for
optimal perfusion of placental bed
Rapid excretion after delivery

7. Muscle Relaxants   *a) Suxamethonium*
2 mg/kg after pretreatment with
20 mg gallamine
b) Alcuronium
Preferred to gallamine (which may
cross placenta) and pancuronium
(which may be difficult to reverse
after short procedure)

	c) Vecuronium
	Muscle relaxant of choice, given using the preloading technique for rapid intubation,
	Short duration
	Prior use of suxamethonium increases sensitivity to vecuronium
8. Oxytocic Agent	*Pitocin*
	5–10 units i.v. at delivery
	30 units in 200 ml as slow i.v. infusion
	Avoid ergometrine
9. Standard Administration Procedure	1. Left lateral tilt on admission to theatre
	2. i.v. line and working suction line
	3. Assistant for anaesthetist mandatory
	4. Cricoid pressure during induction
	5. Routine endotracheal intubation

H. Diabetes Mellitus

Condition falls into one of two categories:
- Insulin dependent
- Non-insulin dependent

and is managed by:
- Diet alone or in combination with
- Oral hypoglycaemics
- Insulin

Oral Hypoglycaemics

Drug class – Sulphonylureas	Dose range mg/24 h
Tolbutamide	500–2000
Chlorpropamide	100–375
Acetohexamide	500–1500
Glymidine	500–2000
Glibenclamide	2.5–15
Glipizide	2.5–30
Glibornuride	12.5–75
Gliclazide	40–320
Gliquidone	15–180

Drug class – Biguanides

Metformin	1000–2000
Phenformin	25–100
Butylbiguanide	100–300

Note: These drugs may cause severe metabolic acidosis during anaesthesia and should be discontinued before surgery.

Drug class – Insulins

Rapidly-acting – 4–6 h:
Soluble insulin of beef or human type (with genetic engineering methods).
Actrapid monocomponent (MC) – pork

Intermediate-acting – 15–18 h:
Semilente (beef), Semitard MC (pork), Rapitard MC (beef and pork), Globin insulin (beef), Isophane (beef), Lente (beef), Lentard MC (beef and pork), Monotard MC (pork)

Long-acting – > 24 h:
Protamine zinc (beef), Ultralente (beef), Ultratard MC (beef)

I. Cardiac Stimulants

Adrenaline/Epinephrine	Standard solution is 1 mg/ml. May be given subcutaneously 0.2–0.5 mg in adults. As treatment during cardiac arrest 1 mg is diluted in 10 ml saline and given endotracheally or intravenously in increments. Otherwise use 1 mg/200 ml i.v. solution as with isoprenaline.
Isoprenaline (Isuprel)	0.8 mg/200 ml saline or dextrose 5% in water as a very slow i.v. infusion.
Dopamine (Intropin)	250 mg/200 ml as above
Dobutamine (Dobutrex)	250 mg/200 ml as above
Glucagon	2.5–5.0 mg i.v. over 1 min; can be repeated hourly or 10 mg/200 ml as above
Calcium chloride	10 ml/kg i.v.

Digitalis	– *Lanatoside-C* 1.2–1.6 mg	i.v. as digitalizing dose.
	– *Digoxin* 0.5–2.0 mg	Acts within 15–30 min
	– *Strophanthin* 0.5 mg	

Note: 1. Dopamine promotes renal blood flow.

2. Dobutamine produces best inotropic effect without tachycardia.

3. Calcium/digitalis drug interaction

J. Suggested Concentrations for Use as Continuous Infusions

	Per ml	Per 200 ml	Dose/min	*Drops/10 kg
Lignocaine	5 ml	1 g	25–50 µg/kg	3–6
Nitroglycerine	1.25 mg	250 mg	0.5–5 µg/kg	from 3.5
Nitroprusside	100 µg	20 mg	from 0.5 µg/kg	from 3.5
Trimetaphan	1.25 mg	250 mg	from 100 µg/kg	from 1.0
Phentolamine	1.25 mg	250 mg	from 10 µg/kg	5
Adrenaline	5 µg	1 mg	from 0.5 µg/kg	from 2.5
Isoprenaline	5 µg	0.8 mg	from 0.5 µg/kg	from 2.5
Dopamine	1.25 mg	250 mg	2.5–20 µg/kg	from 2.5
Dobutamine	1.25 mg	250 mg	2.5–2.0 µg/kg	from 2.5
Phenylephrine	50 µg or	10 mg	50 µg/kg dose, not for pro-	10} single dose, thereafter
Metaraminol	10 drops	10 mg	longed use	1 dr/10 kg/min
Ketamine	2 mg	400 mg	5 µg/kg	1.5
Amrinone	0.5 mg	100 mg	10–30 µg/kg	10–15

Note: Using a microdropper (*60 drops=1 ml) drip rate per min equals volume in ml infused per h.

Drugs for i.v. injection

	Dosage (µg/kg/min)	Concentration	Dilution in 5% dextrose H_2
Dopamine	2–5 (dopamine receptors) 5–20 (beta) >20 (alpha)	1 mg/ml	200 mg in 200 ml
Dobutamine	2–20	1 mg/ml	250 mg in 200 ml
Isoprenaline (Isuprel)	0.02–0.2	2 µg/ml	0.4 mg in 200 ml
Adrenaline	0.005–0.02 (beta) >0.02 (alpha and beta)	5 µg/ml	1 ml in 200 ml

Analeptics

1. *Doxapram* – i.v. dose not to exceed 1 mg/kg. Titrate slowly against response. Strong respiratory stimulant, with arousal, leading to convulsive seizure in overdose.

2. *Nikethamide (Coramine)* – 1–2 ml of 25% solution

3. *Physostigmine* – Central cholinergic drug. Antagonizes anticholinergic agents (scopolamine, phenothiazines, tricyclic antidepressants) and GABA synapse activators (diazepines). Relieves opiate sedative and respiratory depression.
0.01–0.04 mg/kg, up to 0.08 mg/kg. Peak action ± 10 min, duration 60–120 min. May require peripheral anticholinergic block (glycopyrrolate).

4. *Naloxone (Narcan)* – Specific opiate antagonist. Dose 0.0005–0.001 mg/kg. Rapid onset, short duration (30 min). Minimal symptoms with overdose. For longer action use i.m. only; i.v. infusion, especially in neonates, depressed by intrapartum opiate to mother.
This drug supersedes nalorphine and levalorphan.

K. Bronchodilators

1. β-agonists

Agents	β1	β2	Dose
Orciprenaline (Alupent)	+	+ + +	500 µg slowly i.v.
Terbutaline (Bricanyl)	+	+ + +	½–1 tab tds
Carbuterol (Bronsecur)	–	+ + +	2 mg tds
Fenoterol (Berotec)	–	+ + +	1–2 tabs tds
Hexaprenaline (Ipradol)		+ +	½–1 ampoule i.v. = 2 ml = 5 µg
Salbutamol (Ventolin)	±	+ + +	up to 0.5 µg/kg/min

2. Anticholinergics

Inhalation of irritants will provoke bronchospasm in asthmatics; this can be prevented by prior treatment with atropine.

Dose: 0.6 mg slowly i.v. May be repeated up to 3 mg.

Ipratropium (Atrovert) by aerosol avoids all the side effects of parenteral anticholinergics. It is effective at a dose of 100 µg.

3. Phosphodiesterase inhibitions

a) Aminophylline. Loading doses of 6–9 mg/kg intravenously over 10–12 min. Thereafter continuous infusion of 0.9–1.3 mg/kg/h to achieve plasma level of 10–20 µg/ml. Drug ineffective at levels under 10 µg/ml. Side effects at levels above 20 µg/ml.

b) Diprophylline (Silbephylline)
c) Oxtriphylline (Choledyl)

4. Steroids

Valuable in long-term control as well as for acute incidents.

Short acting, from ±0.5 to <12 h	Anti-inflamm. activity	Salt retention	Equiv. doses of glucocorticoids (mg)
Hydrocortisone (Solucortef)	1	+ +	50
Cortisone (Cortogen)	1	+ +	100
Intermediate acting, from ±0.5 to 12–36 h			
Prednisone (Meticorten)	5	+	20
Prednisolone (Meticortelone)	5	+	20
Methylprednisolone (Medrol)	5	0	16
Triamcinolone			16
Long acting, from ±0.5 to >48 h			
Betamethasone (Celestone)	30	0	3
Dexamethasone (Decadron)	30	0	3
Fludrocortisone	15	+ + + +	

L. Growth Charts

See Chapter 4 II. F. for growth tables for infants and children.

M. Common Pharmacokinetic Terminology

One-, Two- and Three-Compartment Models: The decline of drug levels in plasma normally follows an exponential decay, but the actual decay curve is often the sum of two or more exponentials of differing time constants. Normally, a drug is distributed between a central blood compartment and the tissues, gaining access to the blood first. Thus, a two-compartment model is the simplest for practical purposes. Sometimes the distribution of a drug appears to be between three or more compartments – these being body tissues having different affinities for or abilities to degrade the drug, and not discrete body compartments.

First Order Reaction: One in which the rate of change in the drug amount is proportional to the concentration of the drug.

Zero Order Reaction: A reaction that proceeds at a constant rate independent of the drug concentration, so that a constant amount of drug is cleared per unit of time (e.g. alcohol).

Steady State: A dynamic equilibrium in which uptake or input of drug is equal to elimination, resulting in a constant level.

Half-life ($T_{1/2}$): The time it takes for the concentration of the drug in plasma to fall by 50%. This term is applied to first-order elimination, and at least two phases are distinguished: a distributive (alpha) phase from plasma to tissue which is usually fast; an elimination (beta) phase which reflects the breakdown or excretion, is always longer, and is often regarded as the "half-life" in the body.

Apparent Volume of Distribution: This is a way of expressing the extent of distribution of the drug throughout body fluids and tissues as if it were dissolved in water. Often the apparent volume of distribution is greater than the body volume, meaning that there is a higher concentration in body fluids or tissues than in plasma, as occurs with a fat-soluble drug. A small volume of distribution means that the drug is retained in the plasma.

Drug Elimination: The various processes responsible for removal of a drug from body fluids, including renal and faecal excretion, hepatic metabolism, and loss of volatile substances in the breath.

Drug Clearance: A direct index of the elimination of a drug from the central compartment, expressed as millilitres of plasma per minute. A short $T_{1/2}$ is equivalent to rapid clearance.

First-Pass Effect: The removal by the liver of a drug that gains first access to the circulation via the hepatic portal system by oral or peritoneal routes. A large first-pass effect explains a marked difference between oral and parenteral doses of a drug which are equipotent.

Hepatic Clearance: The volume of blood flowing through the liver which is totally cleared in a unit of time. This will depend on the liver perfusion of about 25% of the cardiac output.

Tissue Availability: A drug in the central compartment binds to plasma protein which will influence the amount of free drug available for transfer to the tissue compartment. Binding is again influenced by ionisation at tissue fluid pH. This depends on the pKa of the drug. If this is less than tissue fluid pH then ionisation is promoted if basic, vice versa if acid.

Pharmacokinetics is what the body does to the drug; *pharmacodynamics* is what the drug does to the body [19].

N. Some Pharmacokinetic Values for Anaesthetic Drugs

These values should be taken as rough guides only. Not only is there not always agreement by various authors on their values, but there are also considerable variations based upon renal and liver disease, the degree of protein binding which may be affected by other simultaneously used drugs, and the effects of other anaesthetics on clearance rates.

Drug	Vol. of distrib V_d (l/kg)	$T_{1/2}$, alpha (min)	$T_{1/2}$, beta (min)	Clearance (ml/kg/min)
Fentanyl	4	2–13	219	13
Alfentanil	0.9	3.5–11	94	5
Morphine	3.2	3–20	210	11–23
Pethidine	4.1	4–17	222	11
Tubocurarine	0.61		170	2.9
Gallamine	0.24		160	1.2
Alcuronium	0.32		200	1.4
Atracurium	0.16	2–3.5	20	5.5
Vecuronium	0.27	7:4	55	5.1
Pancuronium	0.31	5–13	116	1.8
Metocurine	0.45		220	1.2
Neostigmine	0.70		80	9.0
Edrophonium	1.10		110	9.6
Ketamine	3.0	15	160	20
Methohexitone	1.15–2.1	5	240	10–12
Thiopentone	1.5–3.3	2.4–3.3	300–700	1.6–4.3
Etomidate	2.2	2.7	60–90	20–26
Disoprofol	4.6	2.5	50	60
Diazepam	0.7–1.7	30–66	24–57	0.24–0.53
Midazolam	1.1–1.7	6–15	100–150	6.4–11
Lorazepam	0.8–1.3	3–10	650–1300	0.8–1.8
Flunitrazepam				
Lignocaine	3.6	57	96	0.95
Mepivacaine	2.5	43	114	0.76
Prilocaine	6.5	29	93	2.84
Bupivacaine	3.5	162	210	0.47
Etidocaine	10	129	156	1.22

From [23, 29]

O. Drugs Influencing Intracranial Pressure

Within the closed cavity of the skull are three major tissue compartments:
- Brain
- Blood
- Cerebrospinal fluid

Changes in intracranial pressure originate in volume changes of one compartment and can be compensated for by changes in the others.

Mechanisms whereby intracranial pressure (ICP) can be influenced, and the drugs acting through these mechanisms, include:

1. Changes in $CMRO_2$ – an increase in rate increases ICP
   Raises: ketamine, convulsants and analeptics
   Decreases: thiopentone, etomidate, alfathesin, benzodiazepines, opiates
   Provided respiratory depression is avoided
2. Fluid shifts into brain tissue – brain oedema raises ICP
   Raises: osmotically active solutes that can penetrate blood-brain barrier, including urea, glucose. Substances causing direct tissue damage or metabolic injury, e.g. hypoglycaemia, hypoxia
   Decreases: substances raising osmotic pressure of blood (urea and dextrose), other diuretics, steroids such as dexamethasone
3. Drugs interfering with circulatory autoregulation – vasodilatation raises ICP by increasing intracerebral blood volume
   Raises: volatile anaesthetics (excluding N_2O), any respiratory depressant through hypercarbia and hypoxia
   Decreases: hypotensive drugs, vasodilator drugs – nitroglycerin, sodium nitroprusside, trimetaphan, some calcium channel blockers, hypertensive drugs
4. Changes in central venous pressure influencing outflow pressure from skull
   Raises: fluid overload, coughing, muscle spasm or convulsions (suxamethonium)
   Decreases: various pharmacological means for lowering CVP, head-high position, and muscle relaxants

Drugs for reducing intracranial pressure

Osmotic diuretics	Mannitol 20%	0.5–1.5 mg/kg (bolus)
Loop diuretics	Frusemide	0.15–0.6 mg/kg (bolus)
	Bumetanide	0.001–0.002 mg/kg (bolus)
	Hydrochlorthiazide	2.5 mg/kg (bolus)
	Acetazolamide	5 mg/kg (bolus)

	Start infusion and titrate	
Vasodilators	Sodium nitroprusside 0.01%	0.2-1.0 μg/kg/m
	Trimetaphan 0.2%	10-50 μg/kg/m
	*Nitroglycerin 0.04%-0.1%	0.2-5.0 μg/kg/m
	Diazoxide	3-5 μg/kg (bolus)
	Chlorpromazine	2.5-5 mg (bolus)
	Hydralazine	0.3-0.6 mg/kg

* Maximum total dose 1 mg/kg

P. Assessment of Neuromuscular Block

The nature and depth of neuromuscular block with curare-like drugs is most accurately assessed using electrical stimulation, and recording the response with a force transducer or electromyographically. Interpretation of the mechanical and the EMG response may differ.

Nature of Block: A depolarising block produces a uniform reduction in contraction force with all types of stimulus.

A nondepolarising block produces *fatiguability* of muscle in response to repeated single stimuli, a *fade* of contraction during a period of tetanic stimulation, and a *post-tetanic facilitation* of contraction force after a rest period following tetanic stimulation.

Degrees of Block: Clinical assessment of the degree of block is best made using a train-of-four (TOF) nerve stimulator which is specific for the effect only of *competitive or nondepolarising blockers*. This produces four stimuli at 2 Hz (0.5-s intervals) every 12 s. A supramaximal stimulus must be used. Absolute force of contraction is less significant than the relationship of the 1st to the 4th response.

Stages of Increasing Block:
1. Initially there is reduction in the force of contraction with little fatiguability – the force of the 4th is at least 70% that of the 1st.

2. The 4th twitch is less than 70% of the 1st –	50% block
3. The 4th twitch is absent	75% block
4. Both 3rd and 4th twitches are absent	80% block
5. Second, 3rd and 4th twitches absent	90% block
6. No response	> 100% block

Note: A 100% block may not be reversible with antagonists.
The aim is to produce a block of between 75% and 95% for abdominal surgery.

Reversability: The deeper the block, the more unpredictable its reversal by neostigmine or edrophonium becomes. A block of 100% (which may represent a gross overdose) will probably not reverse. Reversability becomes reliable when the block is <90%.

The following 2 figures illustrate the use of a train-of-four nerve stimulator in the assessment of the depth on neuromuscular block produced by the competitive or non-depolarizing blockers using a supramaximal stimulus applied through skin selectrodes, generally over the ulnar or median nerves on the forearm or wrist.

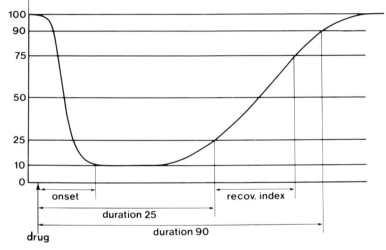

After the intravenous injection of a competitive relaxant there is a delay (onset time), usually of about 5 min, before the full block develops. To be significant for abdominal surgery a block of greater than 75% (25% twitch contraction or less) is needed. On recovery of 75% of the original twitch strength, adequate muscle strength for maintaining the airway and breathing is deemed to have returned. During the 25%-75% recovery, relaxation will be inadequate for upper abdominal surgery and spontaneous respiration will be ineffective.

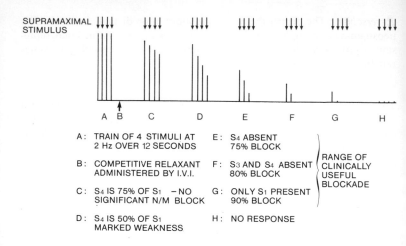

SUPRAMAXIMAL STIMULUS

A: TRAIN OF 4 STIMULI AT 2 Hz OVER 12 SECONDS

B: COMPETITIVE RELAXANT ADMINISTERED BY I.V.I.

C: S_4 IS 75% OF S_1 – NO SIGNIFICANT N/M BLOCK

D: S_4 IS 50% OF S_1 MARKED WEAKNESS

E: S_4 ABSENT 75% BLOCK

F: S_3 AND S_4 ABSENT 80% BLOCK

G: ONLY S_1 PRESENT 90% BLOCK

H: NO RESPONSE

RANGE OF CLINICALLY USEFUL BLOCKADE

Chapter 4

I. Clinical Problems and Solutions

A. Potential Drug Interaction with Drugs Used in Anaesthesia

Medication	Interaction	Potential for occurrence*
Corticosteroids	Hypoadrenalism, hypotension	2–3
Antihypertensives 1. Reserpine, methyl dopa, guanethidine	Catecholamine depletion with reduced sympathetic activity (hypotension); decreased anaesthetic requirement; exaggerated response to vasopressors	1–2–3
2. Nitroprusside, TNT	Hypotension	
Antiarrhythmics quinidine, procaine amide, lignocaine, propranol	Potentiation of muscle relaxant activity, hypotension	2–3
	Severe myocardial depression, atrioventricular block, asthma	1–2–3
Digitalis compounds	Atrioventricular block, ventricular arrhythmias (note: these complications increase with hypokalaemia)	1–2
Tricyclic antidepressants	Decreased catecholamine re-uptake, hypertension, tachycardia	1–2–3
Beta-adrenergic blocking	Bronchospasm with noncardioselective drugs May precipitate acute heart failure: myocardium is resistent to inotropes Adrenaline and noradrenaline produce overriding vasoconstrictor effects – hypertension, bowel ischaemia	
Adrenaline and other α agonists	Cardiac arrhythmias and arrest with cyclopropane, halothane, trichloroethylene, ethyl chloride, chloroform Overriding alpha affects in the presence of beta blockers with unopposed vasoconstrictor activity	

* Occurrence is classified as: *1:* proven in man; *2:* proven in animal; *3:* theoretical.

Medication	Interaction	Potential for occurrence*
Monoamine oxidase inhibitors (MAOI) Ipromiazid (Marsilid) Isocarboxazid (Marplan)	Exaggerated response to adrenergic drugs	1–2–3
Nialamide (Niamid)	Anaesthetics potentiated	
Pargyline (Eutonyl) Phenelzine (Nardil)	Hyperexcitability or coma with pethidine, amidone and other opiates	
Antibiotics Streptomycin, kanamycin Neomycin (aminoglycosides) Polymyxin	Muscle weakness, prolonged curarization Resistant to neostigmine (may respond to i.v. CaCl$_2$)	1–2–3
Anticoagulants Heparin Phenindione Wafarin	Uncontrolled bleeding with nasal intubation Haematomata with local analgesic blocks or intramuscular injections, internal jugular cannulation	
Anticholinesterases Ecothiophate Organophosphorus insecticides	Potentiation of suxamethonium, neostigmine, antagonism of nondepolarizing relaxants Interaction with local anaesthetics and certain antiarrhythmic drugs	
Diuretics Thiazides, furosemide	Electrolyte depletion: (particularly K$^+$ and Mg^{2+}), hypotension, arrhythmias (?? CNS depression and/or convulsion)	1–2–3
Carbonic anhydrase inhibitors	Potentiate muscle relaxants	
Mannitol	Blood volume, electrolyte depletion	
Hyperalimentation regimens (mostly related to 50% glucose)	Hypoglycaemic shock, hyperosmolar states including convulsions	2–3
Insulin	Hypoglycaemic shock	1–2–3

* Occurrence is classified as: *1:* proven in man; *2:* proven in animal; *3:* theoretical.

Medication	Interaction	Potential for occurrence*
CNS depressants Barbiturates, meprobamate, dilantin	Enzyme induction increases volatile anaesthetic metabolism (toxicity?)	2–3
Benzodiazepines: (diazepam, lorazepam)	Atropine-like effects	1–2–3
All CNS depressants	Tolerance to other CNS depressants as in alcoholics	2–3
Ganglion-blocking drugs Trimetaphan Pentolinium Hexamethonium	Curarisation potentiated, pupils dilated and nonreactive to light. Other antihypertensive drugs potentiated	

* Occurrence is classified as: *1:* proven in man; *2:* proven in animal; *3:* theoretical.

B. Causes of Bleeding During Anaesthesia

Anaesthetic Causes

1. Respiratory obstruction
2. Hypercarbia
3. Coughing during induction or maintenance
4. Resistance in anaesthetic circuit
5. Hypoxia
6. Induction; due to vasodilatation
7. Cyclopropane anaesthesia
8. Atropine
9. Injection of the wrong drug

Non-Anaesthetic Causes

1. Venous engorgement: overtransfusion, heart disease, tourniquets, position
2. Disturbances causing increase in basal metabolic rate
3. Operations on vascular tissue
4. Hypertension
5. Systemic diseases, e.g. platelet deficiency, liver disease, uraemia
6. Bleeding due to treatment
   - massive transfusion

- – citrate intoxication
- – incompatible blood transfusion
- – anticoagulants
- – dextran
7. Congenital abnormalities, e.g. haemophilia, decrease in fibrinogen or prothrombin, or factor IX deficiency
8. Severe trauma – disseminated intravascular coagulation

Plasma Coagulation Factors

Disorders of haemostasis can result in either bleeding or thrombosis. Problems may arise with:
1. Platelet deficiency
2. Dilution of clotting factors through infusion
3. Absence of specific clotting factors

C. Treatment of Postoperative Pain

Postoperative pain is acute and limited generally to the first 72 h after surgery. There is considerable variation in the amount of pain experienced; thus, to be effective, treatment must be titrated to the patient's needs. Addiction is not a risk in such short-term opiate use.

Factors influencing severity of postoperative pain

1. Anaesthesia	– Premedication
	– Local or general anaesthesia
	– Elimination times of inhalation agents
	– Intraoperative opiates
2. Surgery	– Site of surgery
	– Nature and extent of tissue injury
	– Duration of surgery
3. Psychology	– Personality of patient
	– Motivation to recover
	– Patient's pain threshold
	– Fear, anxiety, lack of knowledge of procedure
	– Previous experience
	– General psychological preparation of patient
	– Financial problems
	– Fear of cancer
4. Environment	– Single or multibed ward
	– Presence of relatives or friends
	– Attitudes of nursing staff

General methods

Any link in the pain pathway may be manipulated in pain treatment. This pathway extends from the site of injury to the emotional responses and the experience of pain:
- Liberation of tissue hormones, cell breakdown products, inflammation
- Sensitization and activation of mechanoreceptors
- Peripheral nerve conduction
- Nociceptive sorting mechanisms on entry into spinal cord
- Spinal cord transmission
- Primary interpretation of noxious sensation as pain
- Secondary effects of pain experience, e.g. insomnia, depression, metabolic disturbances

Centrally Acting Analgesics

Narcotic Analgesics

Pure agonists:

Agent	I.M. Dose	Duration of action (h)
Morphine	0.2 mg/kg	4
Oxymorphone	0.02 mg/kg	5–9
Pethidine	1–2 mg/kg	2–3
Phenazocine	0.04 mg/kg	5–8 sublingually
Papaveretum	0.4 mg/kg	4
Methadone	0.2 mg/kg	4–9 cumulative
Codeine	0.4 mg/kg	3–4
Levorphanol	0.05 mg/kg	4–6
*Diamorphine (heroin)	0.15 mg/kg	4
MST continuous	0.2 mg/kg	12

(morphine sulphate controlled-release tablets in 10 and 30 mg, each dose calculated to equal 12 h morphine requirement)

* Heroin is 1.5 times more potent than morphine by mouth (10 mg = 15 mg) and twice as potent by injection (5 mg = 10 mg)

Certain analgesics are short acting and have limited application in postoperative pain relief unless given by i.v. infusion.

Fentanyl	1–2 µg/kg	± 30 min – single dose
Phenoperidine	0.02 mg/kg	1–2 h
Alfentanil	4–8 µg/kg	± 30 min
Sufentanil	1–2 µg/kg (post-op. pain)	± 30 min

Narcotic Agonist/Antagonists**

Agent	i.m. Dose	10 mg Morphine Equivalent	Duration (h)
Pentazocine	0.5-1 mg/kg	40	2-3
Butorphanol	2-4 mg/kg	2	3-4
Buprenorphine	0.3-0.6 mg/kg	0.25	6-8
Nalbuphine	0.2-0.3 mg/kg	20	3-4
Meptazinol	1.5 mg/kg	100	5-6
Tilidine	1.0 mg/kg	oral dose	$\pm$ 4-6, variable

** Relative overdoses of agonist/antagonists can be given without serious respiratory or circulatory depression, with consequent prolonged duration of action. Tilidine may produce delayed onset of respiratory depression under such conditions.

All narcotic antagonists except buprenorphine are reliably reversed by naloxone. Tilidine and buprenorphine are absorbed with sublingual administration.

Administration of narcotics: Narcotic control of postoperative pain should aim to maintain constant pain relief without "peaks and valleys" of drug effect. Intermittent intramuscular injection may allow pain breakthrough. Continuous i.v. infusion or intrathecal/epidural injection is preferred. There is a variation of at least $10 \times$ in the analgesic dose of a drug in different subjects depending on pain threshold and endogenous levels of endorphins; thus, i.v. drugs must be titrated.

Morphine 0.5-0.7 mg/kg initial i.v. bolus, followed after 15 min with next titrating dose. Follow-up dose $\pm$ hourly. For continuous i.v. infusion use a loading dose 30-50 µg/kg, with 0.3-0.7 mg/kg/h.

Administered intrathecally, morphine doses of $\pm$ 1-2 mg may give > 24 h pain relief without other sensory loss, but with possibility of delayed respiratory depression. Epidural route is effective; use indwelling catheter.

Keep a pain flow chart with half-hourly monitoring of:
- Patient's pain score (either 10 cm line or "pain faces")
- Blood pressure, heart rate, respiration rate
- Sleep and general behaviour

Such a chart indicates patient response and duration of action.

Nonopioid Analgesics

Ketamine	2-4 mg/kg	i.m.
	0.2-0.75 mg/kg	i.v.
	5-20 µg/kg/min	by infusion

Nefopam	1 mg/kg orally 60 mg = 600 mg aspirin
	0.3 mg/kg i. m. – 20 mg = 12 mg morphine
Nitrous oxide	Inhalation of ± 25% using Entonox/air

Peripheral Analgesics

These are antibradykinin, antiprostaglandin, antihistamine, antileucotrien agents active at the site of injury.

| Lysine aspirin | 30 mg/kg by | i. m. or i. v. infusion, action 6–8 h. |

There are nonsteroidal anti-inflammatory agents in great variety, but oral use is best avoided immediately after surgery. Steroids are seldom used.

Local Analgesics

These are standard local analgesics used in conventional nerve blocks; an indwelling epidural cannula is effective for long periods. Newer agents may become available (e. g. capsacain) that provide days of nociceptive fibre depression.

Cryoanalgesia, freezing a short segment of nerve for 1 min, gives up to 12 weeks of analgesia.

Other Drugs

- Sedatives and hypnotics – benzodiazepines
- Tricyclic antidepressants – can activate adrenergic and serotoninergic descending inhibitory pathways to spinal cord
- Smooth muscle relaxants and antispasmodics
- Antiemetics – domperidone lacks central effects
- Neuroleptics – droperidol, chlorpromazine, sulpiride

D. Transfusion Reactions

Three types may be encountered:
- Haemolytic
- Allergic
- Febrile

A) Haemolytic *Diagnosis* – hypotension, shock, tachycardia, increased bleeding, free-plasma haemoglobin

  Treatment
  1. Stop blood – keep i. v. needle in place
  2. Centrifuge patient blood sample for signs of haemolysis
  3. Send post-transfusion blood sample to Transfusion Service, together with suspect blood pack. If possible, contact the doctor in charge.

4. Insert urinary catheter, collect urine, monitor flow rate
5. Give sufficient $NaHCO_3$ to raise urine pH above 8
6. Give 100 g 20% mannitol intravenously
7. Set up CVP line
8. Infuse compatible packed cells, and monitor CVP to combat shock
9. Do not use vasopressors
10. Approximately 1 h after start of mannitol infusion, give 80–120 mg frusemide i.v. (diuretics too early may "freeze" the kidney)
11. Monitor urine-flow response hourly
12. If signs of DIC develop, consider:
    a) Nonsurgical cases: Heparin 5000 U i.v. stat, and 1500 U at 4- to 6-h intervals
    b) Surgical cases: half above doses (2500 U followed by 750 U at 4- to 6-h intervals)

B) Allergic   *Diagnosis* – allergic skin reactions, pruritis

Treatment
1. Stop blood
2. Promethazine by mouth/injection
3. Bronchospasm treated with adrenaline, corticoids

C) Febrile   *Diagnosis* – pyrexia, sweating, BP maintained

Treatment
1. Stop blood
2. Antipyretics – aspirin or i.v. lysine aspirin
3. Give fluids

E. Air Embolism – Diagnosis

Highly sensitive measures

1. Sudden small decrease in pCO_2 on capnography
2. Appearance of altered praecordial Doppler probe sounds
3. Increased pulmonary artery pressure
4. Aspiration of air from central venous line or pulmonary artery

Less sensitive measures

1. Tachycardia or ventricular dysrhythmia
2. Hypotension
3. "Mill wheel" murmur
4. Increased central venous, right ventricular, or pulmonary artery pressure

Treatment
1. Notify surgeon
2. Compress veins leading from entrance site
3. Lower entrance site (to elevate local venous pressure above atmosphere)
4. Turn patient onto left side in slight Trendelenburg position
5. Discontinue nitrous oxide; give 100% oxygen if possible
6. Aspiration from centrally placed catheter (minimally effective)
7. Vasopressors

F. The Full Stomach

Main problem is aspiration.
Danger periods
1. During induction
2. During anaesthesia without intubation
3. Postoperatively, before full recovery

Causes of vomiting/regurgitation
1. Material in stomach or oesophagus
2. Contents coming from the intestines into the stomach, e.g. intestinal obstruction
3. Delayed stomach emptying
4. Strong breathing movements in the presence of airway obstruction
5. Inflation of the stomach with mask IPPB

Factors causing regurgitation
1. Fluids in the stomach
2. Incompetence of cardiac sphincter; causes include gastric tubes, hiatus hernia
3. Increase in intra-abdominal pressure
4. Subatmospheric intrathoracic pressure
5. Obesity
6. Pregnancy

Dangers of vomiting during anaesthesia
1. Aspiration pneumonia
2. Hypoxia
3. Cardiac inhibition
4. Chemical trauma to the bronchial mucosa, alveolar membrane
5. Airway obstruction

Principles of anaesthetic techniques

1. Decrease the amount of stomach contents – if possible nil per mouth 4–6 h preoperatively. Every patient in labour has a full stomach. To decrease the volume of the stomach contents:
   - let patient vomit – use apomorphine?
   - stomach tube
   - speed emptying with metoclopramide or domperidone
2. Alkalization of stomach contents (but alkaline aspiration syndrome also possible)
3. Avoid general anaesthesia where possible. Use nerve block, topical anaesthesia, neuroleptics
4. Awake endotracheal intubation before general anaesthesia
5. General anaesthetic apparatus – suction, tilting table
- cuffed endotracheal tube – test cuff

Prevention of regurgitation

1. 40° head up tilt
2. Premedicate with metoclopramide
3. Preoxygenate for 3 min together with 20 mg gallamine or equivalent dose nondepolarizer
4. Cricoid pressure by assistant (Sellick's maneouvre)
5. Rapid i.v. induction with anaesthetic and muscle relaxant
6. Do not ventilate
7. Avoid respiratory movements against obstructed airway

Prevention of postoperative aspiration

1. Working sucker, wide bore suction
2. Patient awake before extubation
3. Lateral position during recovery
4. No ventilation without intubation

G. Prevention and Treatment of Aspiration Pneumonitis

1. Assume full stomach when:
   a) patient has eaten within past 6 h
   b) pregnancy (last trimester)
   c) recent trauma
   d) acute abdomen
   e) reflux oesophagitis/heartburn
   f) central nervous system dysfunction (coma)
   g) obstruction of gastrointestinal tract (including peptic ulcers and pyloric stenosis, gastrointestinal bleeding)

h) gastric emptying prolonged by drugs, e.g. narcotics
i) achalasia
j) incompetent swallowing reflexes
k) oesophageal or pharyngeal diverticuli

2. *Management choices include:*
   a) regional anaesthesia
   b) awake intubation
   c) hydrotalcite (Altacite) to adsorb HCl and pepsin as antacid
   d) "crash" induction, to include:
      - metoclopramide or domperidone
      - nasogastric suction (large-bore catheter), remove before induction
      - high-volume suction
      - slight head-up tilt
      - preoxygenation
      - 3 mg curare (or equivalent) and 3-min wait
      - cricoid pressure (Sellick's manoeuvre)
      - rapid intravenous induction with thiopentone or ketamine and full relaxant dose of succinylcholine
      - no assisted ventilation until endotracheal tube is in situ and cuff inflated
   e) Acid and alkali aspiration give equally severe pulmonary reaction. Use hydrotalcite, which is neutral, or clear fluid antacids (e.g. 0.3 M sodium citrate)

3. *Diagnosis of aspiration:*
   a) demonstration of gastric contents in trachea; measure pH
   b) wheezing
   c) hypoxaemia or increased A-a DO_2
   d) chest X-ray – "snow storm" (may be localized)

4. *Management of documented aspiration:*
   a) leave endotracheal tube in place
   b) remove solid material (by bronchoscopy if necessary)
   c) close monitoring of arterial gases
   d) correct metabolic acidosis
   e) O_2 therapy and/or mechanical assistance to ventilation
   f) intensive chest physiotherapy

5. *Regimens producing questionable or possibly injurious effect:*
   a) steroids
   b) antibiotics (except treatment of cultured organisms)
   c) tracheobronchial lavage with alkaline solution (washes out surfactant)
   d) intratracheal $NaHCO_3$

H. The Acute Asthmatic Attack

Many factors may contribute to acute bronchospasm, which must not be overlooked during anaesthesia. These include:

- Mechanical and chemical irritation of the tracheobronchial tree
- High concentrations of drugs in the pulmonary circuit after i.v. injection
- Allergic response to certain drugs
- Pre-existing bronchitis
- Known asthmatic condition
- Substances introduced through the wound during surgery

Any known asthmatic who is not in remission must at least receive active prophylactic treatment before anaesthesia. This will include antibiotics, physiotherapy, and inhalation of appropriate aerosols, along with i.v. fluids if the subject is dehydrated.

In the treatment of the active attack the following are used:

Bronchodilators:
- Aminophyllin 5–7 mg/kg i.v. as a bolus, or 10 mg/kg/24 h as an infusion; dose may need to be reduced when used with $\beta2$ agonists
- Adrenaline by subcutaneous or i.v. injection, the latter using 1 mg of drug (1 ml/1:1000 soln) diluted in 10–20 ml water, initially 50 µg
- $\beta2$ agonists – salbutamol diluted 5 mg/500 ml (10 µg/ml) for infusion at 0.1–0.5 µg/kg/min
- $\beta2$ agonist aerosols
- Atropine may be indicated to reduce bronchospasm attendant on aerosol inhalation

Steroids:

Hydrocortisone 100 mg	intravenously,
Prednisolone 20 mg	repeat if necessary
Betamethasone 3 mg	

Smooth muscle relaxants:
Amyl nitrite by inhalation from anaesthetic circuit; note vasodilator effect

Oxygen by mask or endotracheal tube with IPPV

I. Correct Intubation of the Trachea

Errors in placing an endotracheal tube may be

- Oesophageal intubation
- Right or left bronchus intubation
- Submucous placement of tube on nasal intubation
- Excessive angulation lead to kinking

Points 1, 3, 4, 12, 13, 15, 17 below are indicators of correct endotracheal placement:

1. *Visualize the tube between the cords:* An absolute sign when anatomical landmarks are correctly identified.

2. *Cough on passing the tube:* This generally indicates that the tube entered the cords and larynx. This reflex is not always present if sufficient relaxant or opiate is given.

3. *Fibreoptic laryngoscope passed down tube identifies tracheal mucosa/ rings:* An absolute sign using an instrument that is not widely available, needing skill in its application.

4. *Capnography of the expired air:* An absolute sign provided end-expired pCO_2 exceeds $\pm 4\%$ over at least ten breaths. Prior ventilation of the stomach may allow discharge of CO_2 containing gas to contaminate the first "breaths" after oesophageal intubation.

5. *Air reflux around tube:* Sound of air reflux in oesophagus is said to be "typical" and unlike tracheal air reflux. It is a sign easy to elicit but is not constant. A deeply placed tube in the oesophagus or one with inflated cuff is more likely to blow into the stomach, usually silently.

6. *Air entry into stomach:* With a stethoscope placed on the epigastrium it is easy to detect the entry of as little as 5 ml air into the stomach from a tube placed in the oesophagus. This should be a routine test.

7. *Chest moves on inflation with anaesthetic circuit:* Upper chest movement is typical of lung ventilation, but lower chest movement may be mimicked by stomach inflation or inflation of the lower third of the oesophagus. In the barrel-chested emphysematous patient this sign may be useless. Chest movement during spontaneous breathing should be compared with the movement on manual inflation, and viewed looking from abdomen towards chest.

8. *Auscultation of chest during ventilation with anaesthetic circuit:* Upper chest sounds are more typical of lung entry. Air entry into the oesophagus may be heard as breath sounds, usually with fine crepitations as opposing mucous membranes separate to admit air. Auscultation of the chest before anaesthesia gives a baseline against which to judge the quality of the sounds during manual ventilation. Sounds can also mimic bronchospasm.

9. *Chest compression ejects gas from endotracheal tube:* To elicit this sign compression of upper chest is important. Lower chest compression may displace gas from oesophagus or stomach. A rigid chest makes this test valueless.

10. *Bag moves with spontaneous respiratory movements:* This will indicate tracheal or bronchial intubation, provided a tidal volume of 200 ml or more is present. Violent respiratory movements can ventilate the intu-

bated oesophagus, but the volumes are disproportionately small and show a square wave pattern.

11. *Adequate tidal volume is returned during mechanical ventilation:* This would seem to be possible only when the stomach is grossly inflated or the LOS closing pressure is very low. In both instances the intragastric pressure must be higher than LOS pressure to allow reflux of gas, and should thus be visibly distended.

12. *Lung has different compliance than oesophagus:* Oesophageal compliance is about 1% of lung compliance, limited when a blow through to the stomach occurs at constant pressure. This is unlike lung compliance, which is a straight-line relation between pressure and volume. The feel when ventilating by hand differs with each, although the compliance of a single lung with bronchial intubation may be confusing.

13. *Inflation of the stomach:* Visible distension of the stomach is a late sign of oesophageal intubation or may have resulted from mask ventilation before intubation, making it unreliable unless the abdomen is observed during anaesthetic induction.

14. *Large tidal volume during ventilation:* A tidal volume of 500 ml or more should signify lung intubation, but the return of similar volumes from the oesophagus/stomach has been reported.

15. *Palpation and auscultation over the trachea:* Air movement sounds close, not muffled as it would be if the endotracheal tube were in the oesophagus. Palpation may show that the trachea cannot be pressed back onto the cervical vertebrae when a tube is in the oesophagus (Sellick's manoeuvre).

16. *Colour of patient:* Ventilating the oesophagus or one lung leads to cyanosis. This may appear only after 10 min if the patient was fully preoxygenated before induction.

17. *Condensation of moisture within clear plastic endotracheal tube:* This is said to occur more readily with gas returned from the lung which is fully humidified.

18. *Lateral X-ray of neck:* This would show the position of a tube, but it is not a normally acceptable method of diagnosis.

19. *Passage of stomach tube or suction tube:* Being longer, a stomach tube is more likely to penetrate deeper and produce acid secretions.

20. *Feel of the bag on compression:* Requires experience of the operator, who must compare the feel of ventilating by mask with a free airway with the feel after intubation. Attention is given to:
    - The pressure/volume relation on inflation
    - Stiffness on inflation with a fixed pressure at which large volumes can be inflated (LOS leakage pressure; *LOS* = Lower oesophageal sphincter)

- The feel of elastic recoil in expiration; gas issues from the oesophagus in a short burst
21. *Bradycardia and arrhythmias:* These are signs of hypoxia and can indicate incorrect intubation. A check of correct intubation and oxygen delivery should precede atropine.
22. *Leave tube in situ - ventilate with mask (21):* Using mask and airway, an improvement in ventilation and colour is the quickest test whilst tube is in situ. If in the oesophagus, the tube protects from regurgitation, which is more likely if the stomach has been inflated.
23. *Auscultate the breathing circuit during ventilation:* A useful method when a stethoscope cannot be applied, or in the severely emphysematous patient.

J. Pulmonary Embolism

Symptoms:	Acute chest pain
	Severe shortness of breath
	Syncope
	Sudden death
Signs:	Peripheral vasoconstriction
	Central and peripheral cyanosis
	Tachypnoea
	Tachycardia
	Raised CVP
	4th heart sound
	ECG lead III-Q wave and inverted T wave
	Leads V_1–V_3 – inverted T wave
	30%–40% die within 6 h.
Diagnosis:	1. Symptoms and signs
	Dyspnoea
	Haemoptysis
	Pleuritic pain
	Crepitations
	Split 2nd heart sound
	2. Chest X-ray

Consolidation and atelectasis	47%
Elevated diaphragm	40%
Pleural effusion	28%
Pulmonary infarction	33%

3. ECG – see above
4. Blood gases   decreased pO_2
                 increased pCO_2
5. Enzymes, LDH raised
6. Lung scan
7. Pulmonary angiography
8. Radioactive tracers

Treatment:

1. *Embolism with few symptoms*
   Heparin – 7 days
   Warfarin
2. *Recurrent pulmonary embolism*
   Anticoagulants
   Tying and plication of IVC
3. *Severe embolism*
   shock ⎫
   tachycardia ⎬ requires
   chest pain ⎮ intensive care
   cyanosis ⎭
   Start with 15 000–20 000 U heparin i.v. and then
   60 000 U/24 h O_2
   Analgesics
   Atropine, isoprenaline, vasopressors
   Digitalis, if indicated
   Intubation and IPPV
4. *Massive embolism*
   Shock – hypotension – cyanosis – unconsciousness –
   cardiac arrest
   Intubation: 100% O_2
   To intensive care
   Vasopressors
   – Inotropic drugs
   – Isoprenaline infusion
   Cardiac arrest must be treated in the usual way
   Consider embolectomy
   Streptokinase therapy:
   – Start with 250 000 U, then 100 000 U hourly for
     3 days
   – Follow with heparin and warfarin

Treatment of fat embolism

Commonly related to severe trauma, burns, stress response, lipectomy;
possible relationship to deranged metabolic response

Symptoms:	As above
	Depressed level of consciousness
Signs:	Petechial haemorrhage, retinal haemorrhage and exudates
	Fever
	Dyspnoea
Diagnosis:	Fat globules in urine. Rise in serum free fatty acids and triglycerides
	Blood gases: pO_2, pCO_2 lowered
	P(A-a) O_2 gradient increased
	Platelet, Hb, HCT may fall
	"Snow storm" lung
Treatment:	Immobilize fractures
	Ventilatory support
	Heparin, aprotinin
	Steroids
	Dextrans

K. Respiratory Depression During and After Anaesthesia

During anaesthesia, respiratory depression may result from the normal effects of specific drugs, cerebral ischaemia, drug overdose, hypoxia, airway obstruction and equipment malfunction.

1. Excessive doses of opiates in premedication or anaesthesia, or their interaction with volatile agents
2. Excessive doses of intravenous induction agents
3. Excessive concentrations of inhalation anaesthetics
4. Synergism between above drugs
5. Effects of muscle relaxants alone or potentiated by CO_2 or drugs
6. Hypercarbia resulting from apparatus maladjustment or malfunction leading to CO_2 narcosis
7. Faults with pipeline connections causing hypoxia
8. Airway obstruction
9. Severe hypotension
10. Electrolyte disturbances, especially hypokalaemia with muscle relaxants
11. Paralysing antibiotics
12. Hypothermia below 33 °C
13. Delayed absorption of i.m. drugs in a shocked patient resuscitated during anaesthesia

In the recovery period following the withdrawal of most depressant drugs, respiratory depression has a limited number of causes:

1. Neuromuscular blocking antibiotics used during surgery
2. Incomplete reversal of neuromuscular blocking drugs leading to early fatiguability of respiratory and airway muscles
3. The second effect of fentanyl
4. Reversal of long-acting opiates with shorter-acting intravenous naloxone
5. Respiratory obstruction; mechanical, by secretions, vomiting
6. Hypothermia
7. Severe hypotension
8. Cerebral and pulmonary oedema

L. Malignant Hyperpyrexia*

Diagnostic clues

Nonspecific	Specific
1. Tachycardia and/or dysrhythmia	1. Myotonic response to succinylcholine
2. Cyanosis (in presence of normal FIO_2)	2. Muscle rigidity
3. Flushing	3. Hot CO_2 absorber
4. Tachypnoea	4. Hyperthermia
5. Diaphoresis	

Laboratory studies and monitors

1. Electrocardiogram (note K^+ effects)
2. Arterial pressures and gases
3. Central venous pressure to guard against fluid overload
4. Electrolytes
5. Serum enzymes, CPK, LDH
6. Urine output
7. Temperature
8. Capnography

---

* By G. G. Harrison

Safe anaesthetic techniques for malignant hypothermia susceptible patients

1. Local and regional analgesia
2. General anaesthesia
   a) Premedicate with dantrolene 1 mg/kg
   b) Monitor temperature and ECG ab initio
   c) Safe drugs include:

Thiopentone	Pancuronium
Midazolam	Nitrous oxide
Rohypnol	Neostigmine
Etomidate	
Morphine analgesics	

   d) Avoid:
   Suxamethonium
   Volatile anaesthetics

Treatment

A) Goals
1. Remove cause of hyperthermia
2. Terminate muscle rigor and hypermetabolism
3. Restore normal acid-base state – neutralize metabolic acidosis
4. Meet increased metabolic demands
5. Reduce temperature to normal
6. Prevent complications
7. Screen first-degree relatives for susceptibility to malignant hyperthermia:
   a) serum CPK estimations
   b) muscle biopsy for caffeine and halothane contracture tests

B) Methods
1. Discontinue anaesthesia
2. Give 100% oxygen by hyperventilation
3. Give sodium bicarbonate for metabolic acidosis (the above may constitute sufficient treatment)
4. Cool the patient aggressively with:
   a) external crushed ice and iced i.v. solutions
   b) iced gastric lavage
   c) iced saline to surgical area if a major body cavity
   d) cardiopulmonary bypass (using vein-to-vein technique)
5. Infuse dantrolene sodium i.v. 1 mg/kg/min until there is
   a) decreased muscle tone
   b) decreased temperature
   c) slowing of the heart rate; *failing the above,* infuse 1 g procainamide or procaine in 500 ml balanced salt solution *or* 1 g Solu-Cortef *or* 125 mg Solu-Medrol

6. Maintain blood pressure and urine output with large volumes of balanced salt solutions, furosemide and/or mannitol
7. Treat hyperkalaemia with glucose and insulin if necessary
8. Treat complications such as DIC
9. Contraindicated drugs:
    a) vasopressors
    b) cardiac glycosides
    c) atropine
    d) calcium chloride/gluconate

M. Anaesthesia for the Diabetic Patient

Diagnosis:

Venous whole blood	Capillary whole blood	Venous plasma
Fasting > 7.0 mmol/l	> 7.0 mmol/l	> 8.0 mmol/l
(120 mg%)	(120 mg%)	(140 mg%)
2HBSS* > 10.0 mmol/l	> 11.0 mmol/l	> 11.0 mmol/l
(180 mg%)	(200 mg%)	(200 mg%)

* Two-hour blood sugar screen

Anaesthetic Considerations:
- Pre- and postoperative monitoring of blood sugar mandatory
- Regular checking of intraoperative blood sugar (hourly)
- Avoid both hyper- and hypoglycaemia
- "Normal" blood sugar levels of 4–8 mmol/l desirable
- Preoperative starvation requires cover of i.v. dextrose infusion – duration of action of hypoglycaemic agents is unpredictable

Immediate Perioperative Management:
The properly prepared and stabilized patient should have:
- No ketosis or metabolic acidosis
- Normal urea and serum electrolyte levels with special note of K^+
- Blood sugar level between 5–10 mmol/l
- Normovolaemic – full hydration for stable circulation

Non-Insulin-Dependent Diabetes:
- Before minor surgery with minimal disturbance of food intake, a minimal disruption of routine is necessary.
- More extensive surgery, change from long-acting sulphonylureas to a shorter-acting preparation.

- Biguanides must be stopped and replaced 1 week before surgery.
- On day of operation omit oral drug, check blood and urine sugars
- If BSL <7 mmol/l, no extra treatment necessary.
- If BSL >7 mmol/l, start constant i. v. insulin infusion.
- Postoperatively, give short-acting sulphonylurea with first food.
- Before major surgery it is desirable to change to insulin control about 3 days in advance – the diabetic-like state produced by acute trauma cannot be controlled with long-acting drugs.

Suggested Blood Sugar Control Regimes:

1. The Blood Glucose Sliding-Scale System. Six-hourly subcutaneous injections of insulin are given according to blood glucose levels:

Blood glucose (mmol/l)	Insulin units
<8.0	0
8–10	5
10–12	10
12–15	15
>15	20
Ketones present	add 5 to dose

2. Constant intravenous infusion of insulin + dextrose. The aim of therapy is to maintain blood sugar levels at 10 mmol/l.

Prepare infusions:
a) 20 Units insulin in 200 ml normal saline
b) Separate 5% or 10% dextrose-containing solution

The insulin is administered using a microdrip (60 drops/ml) set according to the schedule: (drops per minute/10 = units per hour)

Blood glucose level (mmol/l)	Insulin dose
>25	3 U/h (30 dr/min)
15–25	2 U/h (20 dr/min)
10–15	1 U/h (10 dr/min)
8–10	0.5 U/h (5 dr/min)

Insulin in saline solutions should be renewed every 12 h and prepared in plastic containers.

Regimes of insulin and glucose must provide additional potassium and magnesium in infusion solutions.

Adult requirement for dextrose is 100–150 g/24 h – the equivalent of 2–3 ml of a 5% solution/kg body wt./h. Maintenance or resuscitation solutions are used as indicated.

N. Delayed Recovery After Anaesthesia

1. Drugs used during operation in relative overdosage, e.g. phenothiazine derivatives, opiates, intravenous and volatile anaesthetic agents
2. Disturbances of physiology resulting from anaesthesia, e.g. severe hypotension, hypercapnia; a hypoxic episode during anaesthesia; acid-base disturbances; fainting in the dental chair; induced hypotension; hypoglycaemia; hypothermia
3. Disturbances resulting from surgery, e.g. shock, metabolic acidosis, fat embolism, air embolism, occlusion of cerebral vessels, operative trauma in brain surgery
4. Incidental diseases; cerebral embolism, thrombosis or haemorrhage occurring during operation; cardiac infarction; hypothyroidism; hypothermia; hypopituitarism; hyperglycaemic coma with ketosis; adrenal insufficiency; uraemia, liver failure; porphyria; starvation hypoglycaemia; malignant hyperpyrexia
5. Drugs given before operation, e.g. MAO inhibitors (with pethidine during operation); sedatives
6. Intramuscular sedatives and opiates in shock patients later resuscitated
7. Failure of reversal of curare-like drugs with subsequent respiratory muscle fatigue and failure
8. Second effect of fentanyl
9. Other causes of coma

O. Causes of Coma

1. Supratentorial
   a) Cerebral bleeding
   b) Cerebral infarction
   c) Subdural haematoma
   d) Epidural haematoma
   e) Brain tumour
   f) Brain abscess

2. Subtentorial
   a) Pontine or cerebellar bleeding
   b) Infarction
   c) Tumour
   d) Cerebellar abscess

3. Diffuse and metabolic

a) Anoxia or ischaemia
b) Blood sugar disturbances (may be alcohol induced)
c) Feeding deficiency
d) Endogenous organ failure or deficiency
e) Ion or electrolyte disturbances
f) Exogenous poisons – alcohol
g) Infections, e.g. meningitis, encephalitis
h) Concussion
i) Carbon monoxide
j) Hypothermia

Check before anaesthesia:

a) History and physical examination
b) X-rays of chest, skull and cervical vertebrae
c) ECG
d) Circulation; establish i.v. line
   Withdraw blood for sugar, urea and electrolytes, blood gases and oxygen saturation, osmolality, calcium, creatinine, full blood count.
   Investigate for presence of toxins, barbiturates, organophosphorus compounds, benzodiazepines, alcohol.
   Blood smear for malaria
e) Bladder catheterization
f) Treat possible hypoglycaemia with 50 ml 50% dextrose.
g) Check airway. Beware of cervical fracture.
h) Recheck for signs of head injury (scalp, nose, ears), hypertension, fundus, neck stiffness (care), CNS localizing signs.
i) Check body temperature.

P. Complications of Local Anaesthesia

General Rules

1. Observe patient for minimum of 30 min following injection/application of local anaesthetic.
2. Monitor pulse rate and blood pressure regularly.
3. Evaluate all reactions, no matter how mild.
4. Be prepared to treat any/all types of reactions.
5. Inform patient of abnormal reaction.
6. Do not exceed the recommended maximum doses of LA.
7. Do not rely on premedication alone to control systemic toxic reaction.

Classification of systemic toxic reactions

CNS

1. Early stimulation – Cerebral cortex → convulsions
  – Medulla
   a) Cardiovascular centre → BP and pulse *rise*
   b) Respiratory centre → rate rise and/or variations in rhythm
   c) Vomiting centre   → nausea and/or vomiting
2. Depression – Cerebral cortex → unconsciousness
   – Medulla
   a) Vasomotor   → BP *fall,* pulse *rise*
   b) Respiratory and/or apnoea → variations in respiration

Peripheral Cardiovascular (syncope)
   a) Heart → bradycardia or tachycardia
   b) Peripheral vascular system → vasodilation

Allergic
   a) Skin → dermatitis, etc.
   b) Respiratory ⎫   picture of
   c) Circulation ⎬   clinical shock

Miscellaneous
   a) Psychogenic
   b) To other drugs, e.g. vasopressors

Treatment of acute toxic reactions
  Clear airway
  O_2 inhalation
  Fluids i.v.
  Stop convulsions – i.v. benzodiazepine treatment of first choice (diazepam, lorazepam, midazolam)
  Raise BP, e.g. with vasopressors
  Cardiac resuscitation

Q. Hypotension and Anaesthesia

Circulation affected by:
  1. Heart: pump
  2. Vessels: ducts
  3. Blood: content
Hypotension can be caused by changes in any of these three factors.

A) *The heart and hypotension*

   1. Inhibition of impulse formation and conduction is caused by:
     a) Decrease of Na^+ in cardiac muscle
     b) Parasympathetic reflexes
     c) Hypoxia and narcotics
   2. Contractility is affected by:
     a) Ca^{++}
     b) K^+
     c) pH increase; pH decrease
     d) Hypoxia
     e) Filling of the heart
     f) Autonomic nerve stimulation
     g) Cardiac pathology

B) *Pharmacology of hypotension*

   1. Anticholinesterases decrease rhythmicity, conduction and contractility
   2. K^+ decreases force of contraction. High K^+ causes:
     a) dilatation of cardiac muscle
     b) cardiac arrest (asystole)
   3. Anaesthetics – general and local are direct myocardial depressants
   4. Narcotic analgetics can cause bradycardia and decrease vascular tone, and thereby reduce venous return and cardiac filling.
   5. Drugs causing histamine release

C) *Blood vessels and hypotension*

   Pathophysiological factors
   1. Decrease of central vasomotor tone, e.g. overdose of general and local anaesthetics; severe pain stimuli, low $PaCO_2$, narcotic analgesics, mechanical irritation (neurosurgery)
   2. Vagal syncope
   3. Toxic and/or anaphylactic shock
   4. Compression of vena cava
   5. Pulmonary and cerebral embolism, air embolism

   Drugs: alpha-sympatholytic drugs, ganglion-blocking agents, sodium nitroprusside, general anaesthetics, opiates, histamine

D) *Circulating blood volume decrease and hypotension is produced by:*

   1. Haemorrhage
   2. Dehydration
   3. Diarrhoea, vomiting, etc.
   4. Metabolic acidosis and sequestration of blood
   5. Severe viscosity changes

6. Rapid decompression of abdominal cavity, e.g. ascites
7. Fluid deficit during anaesthesia, especially sequestration of fluids into the "third space"
8. Diuretics
9. Acute anaphylaxis

R. The Adrenal Cortex and Anaesthesia

Patients are treated with glucocorticoids for:

1. Collagen diseases
2. Blood dyscrasias
3. Suppression of neoplasms
4. Suppression of immune response
5. Miscellaneous: – severe asthma
              – severe hypersensitivity reactions
              – ulcerative colitis
              – sarcoidosis
              – ankylosing spondylitis
              – skin diseases
              – eye conditions
              – nephrotic syndrome
              – cerebral oedema
              – rheumatoid arthritis

Complications:

1. Insulin requirement increased in diabetics
   Therapy may unmask latent cases
2. Old tuberculosis may be reactivated
3. Peptic ulceration: gastric perforation
4. Delayed wound healing during therapy
5. Osteoporosis
6. Myopathy
7. Hypercoagulability, thromboembolic complications
8. Rarely, hypokalaemic alkalosis
9. Suppression of adrenal cortex response to stress of surgery

Patients particularly vulnerable to stress:

1. Addison's disease
2. After adrenalectomy

3. Large pituitary tumours
4. After large steroid doses for systemic diseases
5. Sudden cessation of steroid therapy

Indications for steroids during anaesthesia:

1. Following gastric fluid aspiration (debatable)
2. After cardiac arrest, acute cardiac failure and resuscitation, for control of cerebral oedema
3. Bronchospasm
4. Neurosurgery
5. Shock (controversial)
6. Transfusion reactions
7. Acute hypersensitivity reactions
8. Laryngeal oedema
9. Immunosuppressive therapy after organ transplants
10. To reduce pulmonary effects of multiple transfusion

When to Supplement:

The chief problem is suppression of adrenal cortical response to stress following steroid therapy, leading to circulatory collapse. Assume that steroid therapy for longer than 2 weeks within the preceding 2 months will produce special operative risk.

1. For immediate emergency treatment of shock, hydrocortisone is the drug of choice. Effect seen within 10 min of i.v. infusion reaches peak after several hours. Intramuscularly, hydrocortisone acts within 1–3 h for 2–3 h. Dosage every 6 h.
2. For prophylactic treatment, depot preparations of dexamethasone and betamethasone are valuable. First dose should be given at least 3 h preoperatively. Daily dose based upon severity of trauma for up to 5 days. May need i.v. hydrocortisone during peak stress period of surgery. Treatment must be tapered off, not suddenly withdrawn.

S. Osmotic Diuretics

1. Indications
   a) Cerebral
      - Preoperatively – to improve the condition of a patient deteriorating rapidly with cerebral compression
      - Intraoperatively during neurosurgery
      - Postoperative cerebral swelling

- Head injury
- Neuroradiology
- After cardiac arrest
  b) Medical
    - With cardiac bypass surgery
    - After operations for intestinal obstruction, generalized peritonitis, urosepsis, and other endotoxic conditions
    - After shock
    - In clinical pictures accompanied by haemolysis and haemoglobin-uria
    - Accidental fluid overload
2. Contraindications for osmotic therapy
    - Active intracranial bleeding
    - Severe renal damage
    - Severe hepatic damage
    - Congestive cardiac failure
3. Choice of agent
    a) Mannitol is given as a 10% or 20% solution in water, 1.5-2 g/kg body wt.
    b) Urea: 30%, 1.0-1.5 g/kg; is now seldom used.

T. Porphyria and Anaesthesia

In porphyria, the blockade of one or more steps in the synthesis of haem from δ-aminolaevulinic acid (ALA) leads to the accumulation of interme-diate products, with the production of symptoms which may mimic an abdominal crisis requiring surgery.

Metabolic pathway: The various porphyrias arise from blocks of the var-ious steps along the porphobilinogen–haem pathway.

Precursor	Enzyme block	Manifestation
Porphobilinogen	Porphobilinogen deaminase	Acute intermittent porphyria
Porphobilinogen	Uroporphyrinogen III cosynthase	Congenital erythropoietic porphyria
Uroporphyrinogen III	Uroporphyrinogen decarboxylase	Porphyria cutanea tarda
Coproporphyrinogen III	Coproporphyrinogen oxidase	Hereditary coproporphyria

Precursor	Enzyme block	Manifestation
Protoporphyrinogen IX	Protoporphyrinogen oxidase	Porphyria variegata
Protoporphyrin IX	Ferrochelatase	Erythropoietic protoporphyria

In addition, through a negative feedback pathway haem inhibits the production of ALA from glycine + succinyl coenzyme A by the enzyme ALA synthase. Thus, any block along the synthetic pathway leads to overproduction of ALA as well as of other intermediates.

Tests for porphyria:

1. Acute intermittent porphyria (Swedish type):
   Urine: ALA + PBG
   Stool: −
   (*ALA*, δ-aminolaevulinic acid; *PBG*, porphobilinogen)
2. Porphyria variegata (South African type):
   Acute phase   Urine: ALA + PBG
   Stool: Porphyrins
   Latent phase   Urine: −
   Stool: Porphyrins
3. Porphyria cutanea tarda:
   Urine: Uroporphyrin I + coproporphyrin I
   Stool: −
4. Hereditary coproporphyria:
   Acute phase   Urine: ALA + PBG + coproporphyrins
   Stool: Coproporphyrins
5. Erythropoietic porphyria (Gunther's disease):
   Urine: Uroporphyrins
   Stool: Coproporphyrins
   RBC: Uroporphyrin + coproporphyrin
6. Erythrohepatic protoporphyria
   Urine: −
   Stool: occasional protoporphyrins
   RBC: Protoporphyrins
7. Erythrohepatic coproporphyria
   Urine: −
   Stool: −
   RBC: Coproporphyrin III

Screening tests for porphyria involve testing for ALA and PBG in urine and for porphyrins in urine, stool and erythrocytes.

Urine Tests:

1. Watson-Schwartz Test: Ehrlich's reagent with sodium acetate added to urine produces a purple colour. On shaking with chloroform colour is not extracted.
2. Porphyrins: Urine containing PBG goes red on standing.

Drugs in Porphyria: The following drugs are considered safe:

1. Intravenous induction agents – Etomidate, propanidid, midazolam, diazepam, propofol
2. Volatile anaesthetics – diethyl ether, nitrous oxide, halothane
3. Neuromuscular blocking drugs – suxamethonium, *d*-tubocurarine, gallamine, alcuronium, neostigmine
4. Sedatives – droperidol; phenothiazines – promazine, promethazine, chlorpromazine, prochlorperazine, trifluoperazine; chloral hydrate; benzodiazepines – lorazepam, triazolam, oxazepam, diazepam
5. Anticholinergics – atropine and hyoscine
6. Opiates – morphine, pethidine, fentanyl, buprenorphine, methadone, codeine, propoxyphene
7. Antiemetics – domperidone, cyclizine, meclozine, droperidol, chlorpromazine
8. Beta-blockers – practolol, labetolol, propranolol
9. Cardioselectives – adrenaline, digitalis, dopamine
10. Local analgesics – lignocaine, bupivacaine, prilocaine, procaine, amethocaine
11. Antidiabetics – insulin, biguanidine
12. Antihistamines – diphenhydramine, cimetidine
13. Anticoagulants – heparin, dicumarol
14. Anti-inflammatory – aspirin, paracetamol; prednisolone; indomethasine, mefenamic acid, naproxen, sulindac, fenoprofen, ibuprofen
15. Diuretics – thiazides, bumetanide, acetazolamide
16. Antihypertensives – hydrallazine, diazoxide, guanethidine, reserpine
17. Antimicrobials – penicillin, erythromycin, cephalosporins, fusidic acid, aminoglycosides, quinine, primaquin

By inference, many other drugs in the same groups are probably safe, but have not been tested.

U. Placental Transfer of Drugs

1. *Narcotics*

   All cross the placenta and depress the foetus.

2. *Barbiturates*
   a) Thiopentone – rapid rise to equilibrium within 3 min
   b) Other barbiturates cross placenta with unpredictable variability in the rate of transfer.
   c) Phenobarbitone is used therapeutically to provide enzyme induction in the newborn.
   d) Ketamine – foetal depression is less than maternal.

3. *Tranquillizers*
   a) Phenothiazines – rapid passage; diazepam also causes uterine relaxation, foetal muscular hypotonia, and impairment of temperature control.
   b) Reserpine – association with the respiratory distress syndrome is suspected.
   c) Chloral hydrate
   d) Tribromethanol (Avertin)
   e) Paraldehyde   All cross the placenta
   f) Chlormethiazole (Heminevrin)
   g) Gamma-OH
   h) Hyoscine – depression and tachycardia
   i) Atropine – foetal tachycardia

4. *Gaseous agents*
   a) Nitrous oxide – even after prolonged administration, the foetal blood content remains 50%–80% that of the maternal blood.
   b) Cyclopropane – ultimately attains 80% of the maternal blood content.

5. *Volatile agents*
   a) Halothane – profound uterine relaxation, depresses foetus.
   b) Methoxyflurane – rapid transfer, foetal depression.
   c) Enflurane – used for Caesarean section with good results; more rapidly excreted.

   All volatile agents must be used in minimal concentrations before delivery to improve placental blood supply without compromising uterine tone and Apgar score.

6. *Local anaesthetic agents*
   a) Lignocaine – up to 50% of maternal level may be found in the newborn.
   b) Prilocaine – methaemoglobinaemia has been found in infants.

c) Mepivacaine – up to 70% of maternal levels in newborn are usual.
d) Bupivacaine – reported foetal concentrations are only 30%–40% that of the mother; long persistence due to protein binding.

7. *Relaxants*
   a) Depolarizing agents – no significant transfer
   b) Nondepolarising agents
      - *d*-Tubocurarine ⎤
      - Pancuronium ⎥ These compounds do not cause neonatal
      - Alcuronium ⎥ depression in normal clinical use.
      - Vecuronium ⎦

      - Gallamine – rapid and significant transfer in normal obstetric practice; to be avoided.

8. *Adverse effects of therapeutic agents in the foetus*

Agent	Effect
Hydrocortisone	Cleft palate, mortality increase, later adrenal depression
Prednisone	Promotes aging of the placenta
Sulphonylureas	Hypoglycaemia
Anticoagulants	Haemorrhage, abortion
Antithyroids	Thyroid enlargement
Vit K (synthetic)	Hyperbilirubinaemia
Antimicrobials, sulphonamides	Kernicterus; thrombocytopaenia
Chloramphenicol	"Gray baby syndrome"
Tetracyclines	Tooth discolouration
Streptomycin	Maldevelopment of 8th nerve
Nitrofurantoin	Haemolysis
Reserpine	Nasal oedema
Thiazide diuretics	Thrombocytopaenia
Ganglion blockers	Ileus
Phenothiazines	Thrombocytopaenia, hepatic toxicity

V. Correction of Hyperkalaemia

1. *Normal serum potassium values:*

	ECF	ICF	Body water as % of body mass			
			% ECF	% ICF	Ratio	Total (%)
Adult	3.5–5.5 mEq/l	150 mEq/l	20	45	1 :2	65
Infant	3.5–5.5 mEq/l	160 mEq/l	30	35	1 :1.2	65
Neonate	4.3–7.6 mEq/l		35–40	35	1 :1	75
Preterm	4.6–6.7 mEq/l		50	30	1.6:1	80

Potassium is an intracellular cation and ECF levels are a poor guide to total body status. Hyperkalaemia may result from:
a) Abnormal intake
b) Failure of renal excretion – renal and prerenal causes
c) Acute shifts of intracellular potassium into ECF, usually seen with metabolic disturbances including acidosis

2. *Treatment:*
   a) Physiological antagonism of potassium with calcium
   b) Increase of renal excretion
   c) Promotion of intracellular uptake with insulin + glucose + magnesium
   d) Use of exchange resins

3. *Antagonism:*
   Use calcium gluconate 10% up to 50 ml without dilution, slowly:
   10 ml contains 93 mg (9%) calcium – 4.6 mEq.
   Calcium chloride 10% 5–15 ml slowly; 10 ml contains 272 mg (27%) calcium – 14 mEq. Normal maximum dose 8 g in 24 h.
   Calcium antagonism is the most rapidly effective treatment.

4. *Re-uptake:*
   a) Correct any metabolic acidosis (see above).
   b) Crystalline insulin 10 units with 50% dextrose 50 ml in 30 min (adult)
   c) Magnesium is essential in re-uptake process (1 g = 8 mEq).
   d) Correct other water or electrolyte disturbances.

5. *Renal excretion:* Standard kaliuretic diuretic drugs and mineralocorticoids

6. *Resins:* Kayexelate 15–20 g/6 h orally or rectally

II. Miscellaneous

A. Apgar Scoring

Sign	Score		
	0	1	2
Heart rate	No discernible pulse	Less than 100 beats per minute	More than 100 beats per minute
Respiratory effort	None	Irregular, slow, gasping	Regular, rhythmical, active crying
Muscle tone	Limp	Some flexion of extremities	Active motion
Reflexes	None	Grimace	Vigorous cry, coughing, sneezing
Colour	Pale, cyanotic	Cyanotic extremities	Completely pink

Each "sign" is scored 0, 1, or 2 as indicated at 1 and 5 min after delivery. At 1 min a score of 7–10 is normal; at 5 min a score of 8–10 is normal.

B. Neurobehavioural Assessment of the Newborn (modified from Scanlon et al. [26] and Amiel-Tison et al. [1]

State	
1. Response to pinprick	0 1 2 3
Decrement	No.
2. Evaluation of tone:	
Pull to sitting	0 1 2 3
Arm recoil	0 1 2 3
Truncal tone	0 1 2 3
General body tone	0 1 2 3
3. Rooting	0 1 2 3

State				
4. Sucking	0	1	2	3
5. Moro response	0	1	2	3
Threshold to best response	No.			
Decrement	No.			
6. Habituation to light	No.			
7. Response to sound	0	1	2	3
Decrement	No.			
8. Placing	0	1	2	3
9. Alertness	0	1	2	3
10. General assessment	A	B	N	S

Reasons
Dominant state   Lability of state
Comments

Specific Tests: Responses scored 0–3

Response decrement (habituation to pinprick, Moro response, light and sound)

Stimulus repeated at 5 second intervals until alteration in response noted

Limit number of stimuli to 12 to avoid fatigue

General Assessment: A   Abnormal
                        B   Borderline
                        N   Normal
                        S   Superior

State is recorded before each specific test.

Awake states: A1 Drowsy
                    A2 Awake
                    A3 Bright and alert
                    A4 Intense crying

Sleep states: S1 Light sleep
                    S2 Deep sleep

C. Postoperative Reinfarction Rate After Previous Myocardial Infarction

Various figures are quoted for reinfarction rates and mortality following surgery. To some extent these figures will be influenced by the quality of anaesthesia and perioperative care. Most often cited series is that of Steen et al. [28] with 587 patients undergoing noncardiac surgery.

Time after infarct (mo)	No. of patients	Number (%) reinfarcting	No. of deaths (%)
0–3	15	4 (27)	4 (100)
4–6	18	2 (11)	1 (50)
7–12	31	2 (6)	2 (100)
13–18	30	1 (3)	0 (0)
19–24	17	1 (6)	1 (100)
> 25	383	15 (4)	8 (53)
Unknown	93	11 (12)	9 (82)
Totals	587	36 (6.1)	25 (69)

Of those dying of infarcts, 33% did so within 48 h of diagnosis. In this series 25 of 587 (4.25%) died of reinfarction, whereas < 1% died of other causes. The majority reinfarct within 5 days of surgery, and often this is silent, the symptoms being those of hypotension, pulmonary oedema or dysrhythmia.

Mortality according to age group:

Age	Numbers	Mortality (%)
30–39	10	25
40–49	29	0
50–59	100	2
60–69	223	6
70–79	210	8
> 80	51	9

Various factors will increase the risk of surgery, probably related to the nature of the disease requiring surgery, the effects of trauma, and apparently minor errors of anaesthetic management:

- Surgery on the great vessels, noncardiac intrathoracic, and upper abdominal
- Uncontrolled preoperative hypertension requiring treatment
- Perioperative episodes of hypertension, hypertension with tachycardia, and periods of hypotension

- Duration of anaesthesia has a direct relationship to reinfarction, with an incidence of 17% at 7 h regressing through zero.
- Episodes of hypoxia
- Inadequate treatment of acute pain

Myocardial revascularization surgery appears to decrease the reinfarction risk after general surgery. In a series of 73 patients undergoing 80 procedures, one (1.4%) developed a nonfatal infarction [22]. In another series of 121 patients there was a mortality of 1.7% [4].

The general conclusion is that routine surgery should be postponed for at least 6 months, and ideally for 2 years. Mortality appears to be decreasing through better drugs, monitoring and intensive care techniques.

D. Coma Scales

1. Glasgow Coma Scale

Scoring is based upon the degree of coordination of three motor responses to external stimuli. A low score equates with a poor prognosis.

Observation	Points	Maximum score
Opening eyes:	E	
spontaneously	4	
to speech	3	
on painful stimulus	2	
no response	1	4
Best-quality verbal response:	V	
oriented	5	
confused speech	4	
inappropriate words	3	
incomprehensible sounds	2	
none	1	5
Best motor response	M	
obeys commands	6	
can localize pain	5	
withdraws from pain	4	
flexion with painful stimulus	3	
extension on painful stimulus	2	
none	1	6
Best possible score:		15
Worst possible score:		3

2. *Edinburgh-2 Coma Scale* (E-2 CS; from Sugiura et al. [31])

Scores the best response to maximal stimuli. If the patient scores in the response to questions, no further tests are needed.

Stimulation (maximal)	Response (best)	Score
Two sets of questions:	Answers correctly to both	0
1. What month is it?	Answers correctly to either	1
2. What is your age?	Incorrect	2
Two sets of commands:	Obeys to both	3
1. Close and open your hand	Obeys correctly to either	4
2. Close and open your eyes	Incorrect	5
Strong pain:	Localizing	6
	Flexion	7
	Extension	8
	No response	9
Best possible score:		0
Worst possible score:		9

E. Nomograms for Estimation of Body Surface Area (adapted from Crawford et al. [3] and Talbot et al. [32])

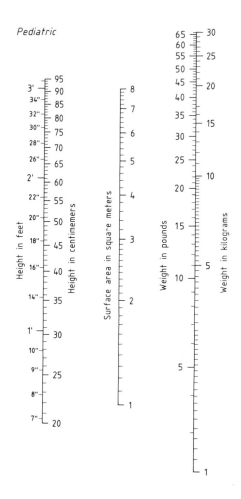

Pediatric

To determine the surface area of the patient draw a straight line between the point representing height on the left vertical scale to the point representing weight on the right vertical scale. The point at which this line intersects the middle vertical scale represents the patient's surface area in square meters.

Adult

Height in feet

Height in centimeters

Surface area in square meters

Surface area (DuBois)

Weight in pounds

Weight in kilograms

F. Growth Tables for Infants and Children

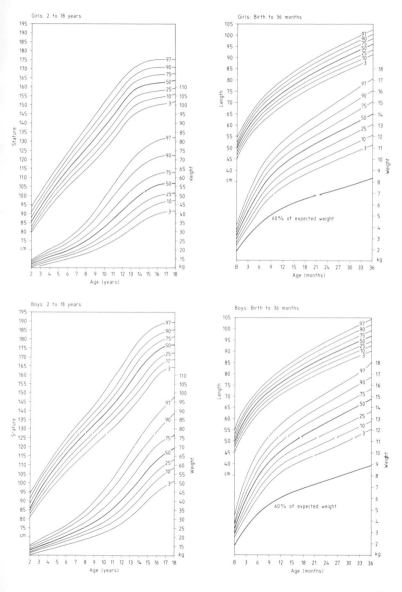

G. Sensory Charts

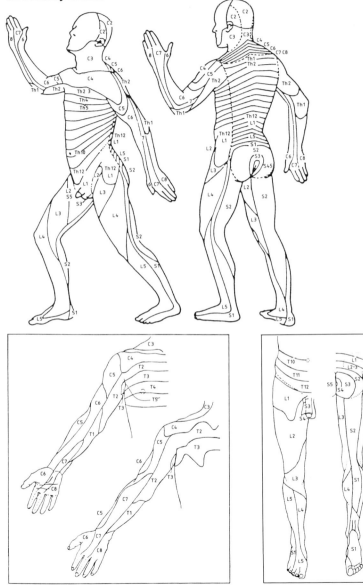

H. Exponentials

There are three common forms of exponential functions:

1. Where the rate of *increase accelerates* with time – "break-away"
2. Where the rate of *decrease decelerates* with time – "wash-out"
3. Where the rate of *increase decelerates* with time – "wash-in"

The uptake and wash-out of volatile anaesthetics and the distribution of drugs in and out of body compartments all proceed in an exponential manner. The rate of change is directly related to how far the process still has to go. Initially fast, it slows progressively until completion. Expressed mathematically, this is the function $y = k^x$, where k is a fixed value "e" = 2.718. At this value the instantaneous rate of the reaction is always the same as the rate of change at that time.

The exponential curve relates the *a* value studied, between 0% and 100% on the Y axis (ordinate) to time on the X axis (abscissa), the time scale being suitably varied. Standard features of the exponential function are:

1. Time constant: The time in which the change between 0%↔100% would have taken place *had the initial rate of change persisted*. In this time a change of 63% does, in fact, take place.
2. Half-life: The time in which a change from 0%→50% or from 100%→50% takes place. Each succeeding half-life, in which a further 50% change occurs, is of the same duration, which is the characteristic of the exponential.
3. The half-life is 69% of the time constant; there are 1.44 half-lives in 1 time constant.
4. The progress of change between time constants and half-lives is:

	Time constant	Half-life
1st	63%	50%
2nd	86.5%	75%
3rd	95%	87.5%
4th	98.2%	93.75%
5th	99%	97%

I. SI Units (Système International d'Unités)

1. Basic Units

Physical quantity	Name	Symbol
Length	Metre	m
Mass	Kilogram	kg
Time	Second*	s
Electric current	Ampere	A
Thermodynamic temperature	Kelvin	K
Luminous intensity	Candle	cd
Amount of substance	Mole	mol

* Minute (min), hour (h) and day (d) will remain in use, although they are not official SI units.

Symbol for "per second" becomes: S^{-1}

2. Prefixes for SI Units

Factor	Name	Symbol	Factor	Name	Symbol
			10^{-18}	Atto-	a
			10^{-15}	Femto-	f
10^{12}	Tera-	T	10^{-12}	Pico-	p
10^{9}	Giga-	G	10^{-9}	Nano-	n
10^{6}	Mega-	M	10^{-6}	Micro-	μ
10^{3}	Kilo-	k	10^{-3}	Milli-	m
10^{2}	Hecto-	h	10^{-2}	Centi-	c
10^{1}	Deca-	da	10^{-1}	Deci-	d

3. Derived SI Units

Quantity	SI unit	Symbol	Expression in terms of base units or derived units
Frequency	Hertz	Hz	$1\ Hz = 1\ cycle/s\ (1\ s^{-1})$
Force	Newton	N	$1\ N = 1\ kg \cdot m/s^2\ (1\ kg \cdot m \cdot s^{-2})$
Work, energy quantity of heat	Joule	J	$1\ J = 1\ N/m$
Power	Watt	W	$1\ W = 1\ J/s\ (1\ J/s^{-1})$
Quantity of electricity	Coulomb	C	$1\ C = 1\ A \cdot s$
Electrical potential, potential difference, tension, electromotive force	Volt	V	$1\ V = 1\ W/A\ (1\ W \cdot A \cdot {}^{-1})$
Electrical capacitance	Farad	F	$1\ F = 1\ A \cdot s/V\ (1\ A \cdot s\ V^{-1})$
Electrical resistance	Ohm	Ω	$1\ \Omega = 1\ V/A\ (1\ V \cdot A \cdot {}^{-1})$
Electrical conductance	Siemens	S	$\dfrac{1}{\Omega}$
Flux of magnetic induction, magnetic flux	Weber	Wb	$1\ Wb = 1\ V \cdot s$
Magnetic flux density, magnetic induction	Tesla	T	$1\ T = 1\ Wb/m^2\ (1\ Wb \cdot m^{-2})$
Inductance	Henry	H	$1\ H = 1\ V \cdot s/A\ (1\ V \cdot s \cdot A^{-1})$
Pressure	Pascal	Pa	$1\ Pa = 1\ N/m^2\ (1\ N \cdot m^{-2})$ $= 1\ kg/m \cdot s^2\ (1\ kg \cdot m^{-1} \cdot s^{-2})$

4. Pressure Measurement, Units and Conversion Factors

Measurement	SI unit	Old unit	Conversion factors	
			Old to SI (exact)	SI to old (approx.)
Pressure	kPa	mm Hg*	0.133	7.5
	kPa	760 mm Hg^x (approx. 1 Bar)	101.3	0.1
	kPa	cm H$_2$O	0.181	5.5

* e.g. BP of 120/80 mm Hg is 16/10.5 kPa

^{x} 1 standard atmosphere = 101.3 kPa = 1 Bar = 14.7 psi = 1 kg/cm^3 = 1000 cm H$_2$O

The litre, though not official, will remain in use as a unit of volume, as will the dyne (dyn) as a unit of force ($1\ dyn = 10^{-5}\ N$).

J. Blood Chemistry Units and Conversion Factors

Measurement	SI unit	Old unit	Conversion factors	
			Old to SI (exact)	SI to old (approx.)
Blood				
Acid-base				
PCO_2	kPa	mm Hg	0.133	7.5
PO_2	kPa	mm Hg	0.133	7.5
Standard bicarbonate	mmol/litre	mEq/litre	Numerically equivalent	
Base excess	mmol/litre	mEq/litre	Numerically equivalent	
Glucose	mmol/litre	mg/100 ml	0.0555	18
Plasma				
Sodium	mmol/litre	mEq/litre	Numerically equivalent	
Potassium	mmol/litre	mEq/litre	Numerically equivalent	
Magnesium	mmol/litre	mEq/litre	0.411	2.4
Chloride	mmol/litre	mEq/litre	Numerically equivalent	
Phosphate (inorganic)	mmol/litre	mEq/litre	0.323	3.0
Creatinine	μmol/litre	mg/100 ml	88.4	0.01
Urea	mmol/litre	mg/100 ml	0.166	6.0
Serum				
Calcium	mmol/litre	mg/100 ml	0.25	4.0
Iron	μmol/litre	μg/100 mol	0.179	5.6
Bilirubin	μmol/litre	mg/100 ml	17.1	0.06
Cholesterol	mmol/litre	mg/100 ml	0.0259	39
Total proteins	g/litre	g/100 ml	10.0	0.1
Albumin	g/litre	g/100 ml	10.0	0.1
Globulin	g/litre	g/100 ml	10.0	
Haematology				
Haemoglobin (Hb)	g/dl	g/100 ml	Numerically equivalent	
Packed cell volume	No unit	per cent	0.01	100
Mean cell Hb concentration	g/dl	per cent	Numerically equivalent	
Mean cell Hb	pg	μ μg	Numerically equivalent	
Red cell count	Cells/litre	Cells/mm^3	10^6	10^{-6}
White cell count	Cells/litre	Cells/mm^3	10^6	10^{-6}
Reticulocytes	per cent	per cent	Numerically equivalent	
Platelets	Cells/litre	Cells/mm^3	10^6	10^{-6}

K. Useful Conversion Factors

Conversion table - apothecary and metric equivalents

1 gram	= 1000 mg	
1 gram	= 15.43 grains	(15)*
1 grain	= 0.065 g	(60 mg)
1 milligram	= 4/65 grain	(1/60)
1 ounce	= 31.1 g	(30+)
1 minim	= 0.062 ml	(0.06)
1 drop	= 1/30 ml	
1 teaspoon	= 5 ml	

* Figures in parentheses are commonly used approximates.

Temperature conversion factors

Fahrenheit to centigrade:
  Subtract 32 from F° reading and multiply by 5/9

Centigrade to fahrenheit:
  Multiply C° by 9/5 and add 32 to result.

Percentage table conversions

0.1% solution	=	1 mg/ml
0.5% solution	=	5 mg/ml
1.0% solution	=	10 mg/ml
2.0% solution	=	20 mg/ml
5.0% solution	=	50 mg/ml
10.0% solution	=	100 mg/ml
25.0% solution	=	250 mg/ml

Solution equivalents

1 part in 10	=	100.0 mg/ml
1 part in 100	=	10.0 mg/ml
1 part in 1000	=	1.0 mg/ml
1 part in 10000	=	0.10 mg/ml
1 part in 20000	=	0.05 mg/ml
1 part in 50000	=	0.02 mg/ml
1 part in 100000	=	0.01 mg/ml

		$\rightarrow$	$\leftarrow$
inch	$\leftrightarrow$ cm	2.54	0.3937
foot	$\leftrightarrow$ metre	0.305	3.28
mile	$\leftrightarrow$ km	1.609	0.62
in^2	$\leftrightarrow$ cm^2	6.45	0.155
ft^2	$\leftrightarrow$ m^2	0.09	10.74
US oz	$\leftrightarrow$ cc	29.57	0.034
UK oz	$\leftrightarrow$ cc	28.41	0.35
in^3	$\leftrightarrow$ cm^3	16.39	0.061
ft^3	$\leftrightarrow$ m^3	0.028	35.314
US gal	$\leftrightarrow$ litre	3.785	0.264
UK gal	$\leftrightarrow$ litre	4.46	0.22
oz	$\leftrightarrow$ g	28.35	0.035
lb	$\leftrightarrow$ kg	0.454	2.205
cmH_2O	$\leftrightarrow$ mm Hg	0.735	1.36
cmH_2O	$\leftrightarrow$ kPa	1.013	0.97
cmH_2O	$\leftrightarrow$ Pa	0.1	10
kPa	$\leftrightarrow$ mm Hg	0.133	7.5

L. The World Federation of Societies of Anaesthesiology (WFSA)

The WFSA was formally constituted at the 1st World Congress of Anaesthesiologists in Scheveningen and The Hague in 1955. Its objectives are as follows:

1. To assist and encourage the formation of national societies of anaesthesiologists
2. To promote education and the dissemination of scientific information
3. To arrange at regular intervals a world congress of anaesthesiologists and to sponsor regional congresses; to encourage meetings of special-interest groups within the speciality and to make provision for them to meet where appropriate at the above-mentioned congresses
4. To recommend desirable standards for the training of anaesthesiologists
5. To provide information regarding opportunities for post-graduate training and research
6. To encourage research into all aspects of anaesthesiology
7. To encourage the establishment of safety measures, including the standardization of equipment
8. To advise, upon request, national and international organizations
9. To apply all other lawful means which may be conducive to the objects of the Federation

The Federation has a President, a Secretary and a Treasurer (the Officers) and an Executive Committee. A General Assembly consisting of official delegates of all member societies is held every 4 years at the time of the World Congress.

World Congresses

1955	Scheveningen	1976	Mexico City
1960	Toronto	1980	Hamburg
1964	Sao Paulo	1984	Manila
1968	London	1988	Washington, D.C.
1972	Kyoto	1992	The Hague

Present officials of the federation are as follows:

President Dr. Carlos Parsloe (Sao Paulo) Brazil
Secretary Dr. John S.M.Zorab (Bristol) UK
Treasurer Dr. Richard Ament (Williamsville, NY) USA
Chairman, Exec. Comm. Dr. Say Wan Lim (Kuala Lumpur) Malaysia

The WFSA also has a European Regional Section and an Asian/Australasian Regional Section, both of which organize international congresses every 4 years, as shown below:

European Congresses		*A/A Congresses*
1962	Copenhagen	Manila
1966	Vienna	Tokyo
1970	Prague	Canberra
1974	Madrid	Singapore
1978	Paris	New Delhi
1982	London	Auckland
1986	Vienna	Hong Kong

The WFSA is a recognized nongovernmental organization of the World Health Organization (WHO), with whom it has worked closely in establishing anaesthetic training centres in Caracas and Manila.

A further project with WHO is the production of a basic anaesthetic manual for use in "first-referral hospitals", and WFSA has also published low-cost manuals on cardiopulmonary resuscitation and obstetric anaesthesia and analgesia.

Currently, a series of books – "Lectures in Anaesthesiology" – is published twice a year, containing contributions by distinguished teachers from various parts of the world.

The WFSA also offers financial assistance to permit visiting professors to undertake teaching visits to developing countries.

Dr. John S.M.Zorab, Secretary, WFSA,
Frenchay Hospital, Bristol, United Kingdom

M. ISO Standards

The International Standards Organization has issued the following list of standards which can normally be obtained from National Standards Bureaux. Lists of national standards are usually more comprehensive than those of the ISO. Those interested should consult British, US, or Canadian standards organizations or DIN specifications.

ISO 4135 – 1979	Anaesthesiology – Vocabulary
	Bilingual edition (i.e. English and French)
ISO 5358 – 1980	Continuous – flow inhalational anaesthetic apparatus
	(anaesthetic machines) for use with human beings
ISO 5361/1 – 1984	Tracheal tubes – Part 1: General requirements
ISO 5361/2 – 1984	Tracheal tubes – Part 2: Orotracheal and nasotracheal tubes
	of the Magill type (plain and cuffed)
ISO 5361/3 – 1984	Tracheal tubes – Part 3: Murphy type
ISO 5361/4 – 1984	Tracheal tubes – Part 4: Cole type
ISO 5361/5 – 1984	Tracheal tubes – Part 5: Requirements and methods of test
	for cuffs and tubes
ISO 5362 – 1980	Anaesthetic reservoir bags
ISO 5364 – 1980	Oropharyngeal airways
ISO 5366/1 – 1980	Tracheostomy tubes – Part 1: Connectors
ISO 5366/2 – 1985	Tracheostomy tubes – Part 2: Basic requirements
ISO 5367 – 1985	Breathing tubes used with anaesthetic apparatus and
	ventilators
ISO 7228 – 1985	Tracheal tube connectors
ISO 7376/1 – 1984	Laryngoscopic fittings – Part 1: Hook-on type handle-blade
	fittings
ISO 7376/2 – 1984	Laryngoscopic fittings – Part 2: Miniature electric lamps –
	screw threads and sockets

Draft International Standards

The DIS number is followed by the expected date of publication as an ISO standard.

DIS 5356/1 86-07	Inhalation anaesthetic apparatus, lung ventilators and
	resuscitators – breathing attachments – Part 1: Conical
	fittings and adaptors for breathing systems
DIS 5356/2 86-07	Breathing attachments for inhalation anaesthetic apparatus,
	lung ventilators and resuscitators – Part 2: Screw-threaded
	weight-bearing fittings
DIS 5369 86-12	Breathing machines for medical use
DIS 7281 86-06	Anaesthetic gas scavenging systems
DIS 7396 86-06	Anaesthetic equipment – nonflammable medical gas pipeline
	systems
DIS 7767 86-11	Oxygen analyzers for monitoring patient breathing mixtures
DIS 8185/1 86-10	Humidifiers for medical use – Part 1: Vaporizers and nebulizers
DIS 8359 86-08	Oxygen concentrators for medical use

N. Setting an Intravenous Infusion

By measuring the time for 10 drops to fall with a given i.v. infusion set, the volume delivered per unit time is obtained. Infusion sets deliver drops of varying sizes, from about 10 drops/ml up to 60 drops/ml. Count 11 drops, the first falling at time zero.

Time (s)	Drops/min	10 dr/ml		15 dr/ml		60 dr/ml	
		ml/min :	ml/h	ml/min :	ml/h	ml/min :	ml/h
5	120	12	720	8	475	2	120
6	100	10	600	6.6	400	1.6	100
7	85	8.5	510	5.5	340	1.3	85
8	75	7.5	450	5.0	300	1.2	75
9	66	6.6	400	4.5	265	1.1	66
10	60	6.0	360	4.0	240	1.0	60
12	50	5.0	300	3.3	200	0.8	50
15	40	4.0	240	2.6	160	0.66	40
20	30	3.0	180	2.0	120	0.5	30
30	20	2.0	120	1.3	80	0.33	20
40	15	1.5	90	1.0	60	0.25	15
50	12	1.2	72	0.8	50	0.2	12
60	10	1.0	60	0.66	40	0.16	10

O. Syringe Coding

One of the common causes of anaesthetic accidents is the injection of the wrong drug. The increasing use of intravenous agents can increase the incidence. One major reason is picking the wrong syringe from a group. People tend to rely on colour or pattern recognition rather than handwritten labels. A code of practice has thus been proposed in the USA (L. Rendell-Baker) and South Africa (SABS 0207 – 1985) for syringe labels:

Standard label size   35 mm × 15 mm

Coding system   a) Upper half coloured according to general drug class
   b) Name of drug overprinted on colour in black
   c) Separate group in a general class identified by white overprinting of colour, e.g. suxamethonium vs alcuronium
   d) Antagonists indicated by diagonal white/colour stripes
   e) Drug concentration indicated on lower part of label – mg/ml

Colour code	Intravenous anaesthetics	Canary yellow	C 61
	Muscle relaxants	Poppy red	A 14
	Narcotics	Cornflower blue	F 29
	Sympathomimetics	Turquoise blue	E 18
	Sedatives/tranquillizers	Light orange	B 26
	Local anaesthetics	Jacaranda	F 18
	Anticholinergics	Lime green	H 41
	Antiemetics	Ash gray	G 26
	Analeptics	Mushroom	A 59
	Unallocated	Wedgewood blue	F 59
		Golden brown	B 13
		Salmon pink	F 57

Label type: Helvetica Condensed ≥ 3 mm high

P. Simple Hand-Held Computer Programs

The majority of readers will have little understanding of computer programming, but can use the computing ability of hand-held units in everyday operating room and intensive care routines. There are several small models available which are programmable in BASIC (of which there are dialects). The simple programs that follow are written for the SHARP PC 1500, 1500A, 1600, and its printer; they are also available under other trademarks. The programs are easily adaptable to other computers using BASIC.

The SHARP applications manual contains statistical programs, stop watch and timer programs, and a program that may be used to test reaction time and motor coordination during anaesthetic recovery (mole banging).

In the listings that follow, $<LN:>$ signifies a new line number that must be entered by the user in an ascending sequence; usually steps of 5 or 10 are used between numbers, e.g. 10, 20, 30, 40, etc. Where a line number is an address referred to in another part of the program, it is given a number – L1, L2, etc. The input of data into these programs follows the commands $<INPUT>$ or $<INKEY\$>$: after $<INPUT>$ the data is first displayed on the screen and entered by pressing $<ENTER>$, whereas with $<INKEY\$>$ the data is immediately entered. Refer to the user's manual of your machine for details of entering and running programs.

1. *Deriving body surface area (BSA).* This program uses the Du Bois equation, given elsewhere in this book, for adults [6] and for infants and small children [10].

$(BSA = kg \cdot 0.5378 \cdot cm \cdot 0.3964 \cdot 0.024265)$.

The address "A" is given to the program.

```
LN:    "A":CLEAR:WAIT 200:PAUSE "Body surface area"
L1·:   INPUT "Ht cm?"; H, "Wt kg?"; W, "Age?"; Y, "Sex M/F?"; S$
LN:    IF H*W*Y > 1 GOTO L2
LN:    PAUSE "Incomplete data input":GOTO L1
L2·:   A = H ^ 0.725*W ^ 0.425*71.84*10 ^ -4
LN:    IF A > 0.7 PAUSE "BSA Du BOIS",:GOTO LN3
LN:    A = W ^ 0.5378*H ^ 0.3984*0.024265
LN:    PAUSE "BSA (paed)",
L3·:   PRINT USING "# #, # #"; A;" sq.m."
```

(This value A can be fed to other programs that use a BSA figure.)

```
LN:    EN
```

2. *Deriving Ventilation volume.* This can be determined from BSA assuming that oxygen consumption is 136 ml/m^2 at 37 °C, that minute volume can be derived from oxygen consumption and a target expired pCO_2. A minute volume is derived based on maintaining a constant expired pCO_2 in the presence of adequate oxygen. The fractional increase of basal metabolic rate (BMR) above 37 °C is taken as 8% per degree (LN+), and as 7.5% below 37 °C (LN−).

The address "V" is given.

```
LN:    CLS:PAUSE "Set Ventilator"
LN:    INPUT "Temp C?"; T, "Desired peCO2?";G
LN:    N = 37-T
LN:    VO = A*136  (A = BSA derived from L4 in program 1)
LN:    IF N = 0 GOTO L6
LN:    IF N < 0 GOTO L5
LN:    FOR I = 1 TO N
LN−:   VO = VO*0.925
LN:    NEXT I
LN:    GOTO L6
L5·:   FOR I = 1 TO −N
LN+:   VO = VO*1.08
LN:    NEXT I
L6·:   MV = VO*0.14/G
LN:    PAUSE "Minute volume",
       LN:PRINT USING "# # #.# #";MV;"l/min"
LN:    END
```

3. This program uses the Radford nomogram to *derive a minute volume and respiratory rate* by "drawing a horizontal line" across the nomogram at a selected body weight. Using the derived minute volume other breathing rate/tidal volume combinations can be chosen. The following symbols are used: *TV*, tidal volume; *RR*, respiratory rate. Leave the program by entering a respiratory rate of 0.

The address "G" is given.

```
LN:   "G":CLEAR:WAIT 150:PRINT "RADFORD NOMOGRAM"
LN:   INPUT "Select body wt kg";W
LN:   TV=2.7476+8.0305*W
LN:   RR=7.5393+103.2556/W
LN:   WAIT 250:PRINT USING "#####.#"; "Tidal volume";
      TV; "ml"
LN:   PRINT "frequency";RR;"min"
LN:   MV=TV·RR/1000
LN:   PRINT "Minute volume";MV;"l/min"
LN:   INPUT "New rate?";NR:GOTO L7
L8·:  PRINT "New TV"; MV/NR·1000;"ml at";NR
LN:   INPUT "Another rate?";NR
L7·:  IF NR>4 AND NR<=40 GOTO L8
LN:   END
```

4. A program for *entering the date and time* on any printed material. It is accessed from the program being printed by the GOSUB command, and returns to the same program. There is no address given here; address the first program line you allocate to this small program. For this to run you must enter the current date and time into the memory by typing:

TIME=MMDDHH.MMSS <RETURN>

using a 0 prefix to single figure entries (e.g. 2nd January at 11 o'clock exactly would be 010211.0000).

```
LN:   CLEAR:A=TIME
LN:   A$=STR$ A
LN:   IF TIME >99999THEN L8
LN:   A$="0"+A$
L8·:  M$=LEFT$ (A$,2)
LN:   D$=MID$ (A$,3,2)
LN:   H$=MID$ (A$,5,2)
LN:   DS$=D$+"/"+M$+"/86" ···(You must set the year – here '86')
LN:   O$=MID$ (A$,8,2)
LN:   T$=H$+":"+O$
LN:   LPRINT DS$+"@"+T$
LN:   RETURN
```

5. This program uses the data obtained from a Swan Ganz catheter to *calculate the derived parameters,* and to print them if required. The printed slip includes the date and time, thus giving the sequence when a number of results are obtained from one patient. Actual line numbers are used because of its complexity. *WL* and *WR* are calculations of the work of the left and right heart.

The address is given as "S".

```
 10:  "S":CLEAR:PAUSE "SWAN GANZ"
 20:  INPUT "NAME";N$,"Initials";C$,"Hosp No";H$, "Birthyear";Y
 30:  INPUT "Ht cm"; L, "Kg"; W
 40:  WAIT 150:PRINT "Your data:"; N$+" "+C$
 50:  PRINT "No"; H$; Y; L; W · · · (If data incorrect press
       <BREAK>.)
 60:  BS = L ^ 0.725*W ^ 0.425*71.84*10 ^ −4
 70:  PAUSE "BSA (C)",:PRINT USING "#####.##"; BS
 80:  INPUT "Qt"; BB, "Heart Rate"; BC, "BP(mean)"; BD,
 85:  INPUT "PA(mean)"; BE, "PAWP"; BF, "CVP (cm H20)"; BG
 90:  B1 = BB/BS:B2 = BB/BC*1000:B3 = B2/BS:B7 = (BE − BF)*
       80/BB
100:  B4 = 1.36*(BD − BF)/B3*100:B5 = 1.36*(BE − BG)/B3*100
110:  B6 = (BD − BG)*80/BB:B8 = B1/BF*1000:B9 = B1/BG*1000
120:  WAIT 0:PRINT "Print out data? Y/N"
130:  A$ = INKEY$:IF A$ = "" THEN 120
140:  IF A$ = Y THEN 290
150:  WAIT 200
160:  PAUSE "CI",:PRINT B1
170:  PAUSE "SV",:PRINT B2
180:  PAUSE "SI",:PRINT B3
190:  PAUSE "LVSWI",:PRINT B4
200:  PAUSE "RVSWI",:PRINT B5
210:  PAUSE "TPR",:PRINT B6
220:  PAUSE "PVR",:PRINT B7
230:  PAUSE "WL",:PRINT B8
240:  PAUSE "WR",:PRINT B9
250:  WAIT 0:PRINT "(R)epeat or (E)nd?"
260:  B$ = INKEY$:IF B$ = "" THEN 250
270:  IF B$ = "R" THEN 40
280:  GOTO 460
290:  CSIZE 2:COLOR 0:TEXT LPRINT C$+" "+N$
300:  LF 1:LPRINT "Hosp no:"; H$
310:  LPRINT "Age"; 1986-Y;" Yrs." · · · (Set current year)
```

```
320:    GOSUB xxxx  ···(Here indicate line number you have allocated to
        program 4 for printing date and time)
330:    LPRINT "BSA"; BS: LPRINT "Qt"; BB
340:    LPRINT "CI"; B1
350:    LPRINT "SV"; B2
360:    LPRINT "SI"; B3
370:    LPRINT "LVSWI"; B4
380:    LPRINT "RVSWI"; B5
390:    LPRINT "TPR"; B6
400:    LPRINT "PVR"; B7
410:    LPRINT "WL"; B8
420:    LPRINT "WR"; B9
430:    LF 2: GRAPH: LINE (20,0)–(210,50)1,0,B
440:    TEXT: CSIZE 1: TAB 25: LPRINT "SIGNATURE"
450:    GOTO 250
460:    END
```

6. A programme using Antoine numbers to *derive the vapour pressure of
water and anaesthetics* at a given temperature [25]. Line numbers are again
included. Data lines are written in sequence: drug name; mol. wt.; density
of liquid; minimum alveolar concentration (MAC) value; Antoine numbers A, B, C. The programme allows a single value to be determined
(Range = 0, Interval = 0), or a series of values from which a vapour pressure vs temperature curve can be drawn. For this a starting temperature is
entered, thereafter the range of temperature, either increasing (+) or
decreasing (−), with the intervals also either (+) or (−), at which the data
points are to be calculated. Knowing the vapour pressure allows the calculation of the usage of liquid anaesthetic drug at a given flow rate. In this programme the delivered concentration is taken as the MAC for the drug.

An address of "Z" is assigned.

```
 10:    "Z": CLEAR: WAIT 170
 20:    "VH": DATA "Halothane", 197.4, 1.86, 0.74, 6.768, 1043.7, 218.3
 30:    "VN": DATA "Ethrane", 184.5, 1.52, 1.68, 6.988, 1107.8, 213.1
 40:    "VF": DATA "Forane", 184.5, 1.49, 1.15, 5.698, 536.5, 141.0
 50:    "VE": DATA "Ether", 74.1, 0.72, 1.94, 7.0268, 1109.58, 233.15
 60:    "VW": DATA "Water", 18, 1, 0, 8.043, 1717, 232.5
 70:    "VP": DATA "Penthrane", 165, 1.42, 0.16, 7.082, 1336.6, 213.5
 80:    PRINT "Vapour pressures"
 90:    PAUSE "(H)alo. Ethra(N)e (E)ther"
100:    PAUSE "(W)ater (F)orane (P)enthr."
110:    WAIT 0: PRINT "Select one: H, N, F, E, P, W"
115:    V$ = INKEY$: IF V$ = "" THEN 110
```

```
120:    IF V$ = "H" RESTORE "VH"
130:    IF V$ = "N" RESTORE "VN"
140:    IF V$ = "F" RESTORE "VF"
150:    IF V$ = "E" RESTORE "VE"
160:    IF V$ = "W" RESTORE "VW"
170:    IF V$ = "P" RESTORE "VP"
180:    READ N$, W, D, M, A, B, C
190:    INPUT "Temp?"; T, "Range?"; U, Intervals?"; S
195:    R = T + U : IF S = 0 LET S = 1
200:    FOR T = T TO (T + U) STEP U
205:    PAUSE "T = "; T
210:    P = A − (B/(T + C))
220:    WAIT 200:PRINT USING " # # # # #.# # "; N$ + "V.P. = ";
        10*P; "mm Hg"
230:    PK = (A − 0.87615) − B/(T + C)
240:    PRINT N$ + "V.P. = "; 10*PK; "kPa"
250:    IF PK < 2.006 THEN GOTO 260
260:    PRINT "Exceeds B.P."
270:    IF T = R THEN GOTO 290
280:    IF T < > R NEXT T
290:    PAUSE "Completed" : PRINT "LIQUID USAGE"
300:    INPUT "Fresh gas flow l/min?"; F
310:    INPUT "Temp"; TC
320:    GL = W/(22.4*(TC + 273)/273)
330:    ML = GL/D
340:    WAIT 150:PRINT N$ + "gm/l gas"; GL
350:    PRINT N$; ML + "ml/l gas"
360:    HL = ML*(F*M*0.6)
370:    PRINT "MAC" + N$; M; "%"
380:    PRINT "1 MAC at"; F; "l/min"
390:    PRINT HL; "ml/hr liquid"
400:    WAIT 0 : PRINT "(R)epeat/(Q)uit?"
410:    R$ = INKEY$ : IF R$ = "" then 400
420:    IF R$ = "R" GOTO 300
430:    END
```

7. A programme giving *dilutions and drip rates* of potent drugs in IV infusions in 60 drops per ml giving sets. Doses are calculated on a body weight basis. The data lines are written in the sequence: drug name; mg to dissolve in 200/250 ml solution; starting dose (µg/kg/min); normal maximum dose (µg/kg/min); loading dose. The abbreviations NNP and TNT are for sodium nitroprusside and nitroglycerine, along with lignocaine, ketamine and adrenaline.

An address of "D" is assigned.

```
 10:   "D":WAIT 150:PRINT "IV drugs by microdrip"
 20:   INPUT "Wt kg"; W
 30:   WAIT 200:PRINT "DOBUTREX=1, NNP=2, TNT=3"
 40:   PRINT "ADREN.=4, LIGNO=5, KET.=6"
 50:   PRINT "ATRACURIUM=7, VECURONIUM=8"
 60:   WAIT 0:PRINT "Select drug No."
 70:   V$=INKEY$:IF V$="" GOTO 60
 80:   IF V$=1 RESTORE "XA"
 90:   IF V$=2 RESTORE "XB"
100:   IF V$=3 RESTORE "XC"
110:   IF V$=4 RESTORE "XD"
120:   IF V$=5 RESTORE "XE '
130:   IF V$=6 RESTORE "XF"
140:   IF V$=7 RESTORE "XG"
150:   IF V$=8 RESTORE "XH"
160:   "XA":DATA "DOBUTREX", 250, 0.5, 10, 0
170:   "XB":DATA "NNP", 40, 0.2, 0.5, 0
180:   "XC":DATA "TNT", 20, 0.2, 3, 0
190:   "XD":DATA "ADRENALINE", 2, 0.02, 0.05, 0
200:   "XE":DATA "LIGNOCAINE", 1000, 25, 50, 2
210:   "XF":DATA "KETAMINE", 1000, 20, 40, 2
220:   "XG":ATA "TRACRIUM", 150, 4, 8, 0.3
230:   "XH":DATA "NORCURON", 20, .7, 1, 0.05
240:   READ A$, S, T, U, L
250:   WAIT 200:PRINT A$; S; "mg/200 ml"
260:   PRINT "Dose"; T; "to"; U; "µg/kg/min"
270:   IF L>0 THEN GOTO 290
280:   PRINT "No loading dose"
290:   LD=L*W:PRINT "Loading dose="; LD; "mg"
300:   PRINT "Drip rate from"; INT (W*T)/(S*5)·60; "min"
310:   PRINT "up to"; INT (W*U)/(S*5)·60; "min"
320:   INPUT "Dose from drip rate?"; DR
330:   DD=(DR/60)*(S*5)/W
340:   PRINT USING "# # # # #.# #"; DD; "µg/kg/min"
350:   WAIT 0:PRINT "(R)epeat/(Q)uit?"
360:   R$=INKEY$:IF R$="" GOTO 350
370:   IF R$="Q" GOTO 400
380:   INPUT "Change wt. Y/N?"; Y$
390:   IF Y$="Y" GOTO 20:IF Y$="N" GOTO 30
400:   CLEAR:END
```

8. A programme for *calculating parameters when using cardiopulmonary bypass*. Calculations are based mainly on BSA so that this programme may be linked to no. 1 above using that data for age and sex. With further data input of pre-bypass (Hct) haematocrit and machine prime volume (clear fluid and blood), it is possible to predict the post-bypass Hct and the effect that a unit of blood would have in raising the level: it is not possible to predict the volume of blood that must be transfused for full correction of the Hct without taking other variables into account. Hypokalaemia is sometimes a problem during cardiopulmonary bypass, and thus there is provision for calculating what a safe bolus of 15% potassium chloride (2 mEq/ml) would be, based upon its dilution in the combined patient and machine blood volumes. The user must decided by how many mEq/l the serum level must be raised, possibly taking the upper limit of normal (approx. 6 mEq/l) as a target. This is not a measure of the potassium deficit, meaning that such a bolus may have to be repeated. The standard calculation for the correction of metabolic acidosis is included. The programme is written so that it stops whenever a result is presented. To move to the next step, press <ENTER>.

The label "H" is used.

LN: "H":CLEAR:PAUSE "Heart lung parameters"
(The next line requests input of data that is already available in programme 1. It can be omitted if linked to it as indicated below.)
LN: INPUT "BSA"; A, "Wt kg"; W, "Age"; Y, "Sex M/F"; S$
· · · · · · ·   *link from here onwards with program 1 or 1+2*   · · · · · · ·
LN: C = A*9E3
LN: PAUSE "Heparin",: PRINT INT C; "units"
LN: USING "# # # # . # #"
LN: D = A*2.5:PAUSE "H.L. flow",: PRINT D; "l/min"
LN: IF Y < 10 THEN GOTO L1
LN: IF S$ = "F" THEN GOTO L2
LN: V = A*2.2566:GOTO L3
L2·:   V = A*2.245:GOTO L3
L1·:   IF Y < = 1 THEN LET V = W*0.09:GOTO L3
LN: IF Y > 1 THEN LET V = W*0.08:GOTO L3
L3·:   PAUSE "Blood vol",: PRINT V; "litres"
LN: Q = V*150:PAUSE "Critical loss",: PRINT INT Q; "ml"
LN: IF Y < 10 THEN LET M = W*4:GOTO L4
LN: M = W*1.5
L4·:   PAUSE "Maintenance",: PRINT INT M; "ml/hr"
LN: USING "# # # # # . # #":INPUT "Hct %?"; J, "Blood loss ml?"; K, "Prime vol L?"; P

```
LN:   INPUT " Prime blood L"; U
LN:   Z—(J*(V—K*.001)+(U*34.4)/(P+V)
LN:   PRINT "Post B—P Hct"; Z
LN:   WAIT 125: PRINT "Restore Hct after bypass"
LN:   INPUT "Present Hct?"; JJ
LN:   JN=(V*JJ+20)/(V+0.5)*0.1: JT=JJ+JN
LN:   PRINT USING " # # # #.#"; JN; "% rise per unit blood"
LN:   WAIT: PRINT "New Hct"; JT; "%"
LN:   INPUT "Base deficit mEq?"; 0
LN:   BE=O*W*.3
LN:   PAUSE "Correction",: PRINT BE; "mEq"
LN:   INPUT "Hypokalaemia? mEq/l"; KK
LN:   KL=KK*(V+P)
LN:   PAUSE "Use 15% KCl bolus";: PRINT KL/2; "ml"
LN:   EN
```

9. *A running clock programme* that updates each second. The TIME string must have been entered.

The label "K" is used: pressing "K" whilst running ends the program.

```
LN:   "K": CLS: WAIT 100
L5·:  A$=STR$ TIME
LN:   IF A$ > 99999 THEN L6
LN:   A$ = "0" + A$
L6·:  M$=LEFT$ (A$, 2)
LN:   D$=MID$ (A$, 3, 2)
LN:   H$=MID$ (A$5, 2)
LN:   DS$=M$+ "/" + D$ + "/86"
LN:   DS=VAL (M$+D/+ "00")
LN:   PRINT DS$
L8·:  T=TIME—DS
LN:   IF T> = 1 THEN L7
LN:   T=T+12
L7·:  IF T>23.5959 GOTO L5
LN:   CURSOR 18: PRINT USING " # # #.# # # #"; T
LN:   WAIT 0: PRINT DS$, T
LN:   K$=INKEY$: IF K$ = "K" THEN END
LN:   GOTO L8
```

10. Patients vary in their response to full doses of heparin (2–3 mg·kg^{-1}). Using the accelerated clotting time (ACT) in seconds as a measure of the anticoagulant effect of heparin, the response of a given dose can be quantified (s/mg per kg dose) for individual patients in order to predict follow-

up doses. The user defines a heparin dose based on body weight. An "ideal" target ACT is taken as 450 s, and the program offers a supplement if this is not reached with the original bolus, based on a figure for heparin "activity" in the patient. On the assumption that heparin breakdown follows a single compartment exponential, and using the peak ACT, the next ACT reading and the time to this reading from the initial bolus, a "half-life" of heparin activity is calculated. Finally, by calculating the heparin activity at a given ACT reading, a neutralizing dose of protamine of 0.6 mg per mg heparin is calculated. This is less than the 1.0–2.0 mg per kg sometimes recommended, but found to give accurate reversal in the authors' hands. These concepts are described by Bull et al. [2]. There is an option to repeat the top up heparin doses using data already in the programme which can also be entered at hourly intervals. This is done by leaving the computer to switch off automatically. It later switches on at the same program step. This program has been written to run with the Time Lapse Program no. 12 so that by entering the time of the initial heparin dose and two subsequent times, the half-life of heparin and the total time of heparinization will be calculated and printed out. This may be left out without affecting the running. Finally, the results may be printed out with name, date and time.

The program address is given as "C".

```
LN:   "C":CLEAR:PAUSE "HEPARIN DOSAGE"
LN:   INPUT "Weight (kg)"; W
LN:   INPUT "Initial ACT (s)"; X0
LN:   INPUT "Heparin dose (mg/kg)"; Y1
LN:   PRINT "Dose (U)"; Y1*W*100
LN:   INPUT "Dose given (U)"; U:Y1 = U/W*100
LN:   INPUT "Time given"; ST$
LN:   INPUT "ACT after Heparin"; X1
LN:   M1 = (X1 − X0)/Y1
LN:   PRINT USING " # # # # # # ."; "Activity"; M; "s/mg/kg"
LN:   WAIT 150
LN:   IF X1 > = 450 LET M = M1:GOTO L2
LN:   PRINT "ACT < 450 - give extra   "
LN:   PAUSE "Heparin",:PRINT ((450 − X1)/M)*W*100; "units"
LN:   Y2 = (450 − X1)/M1
LN:   INPUT "New ACT?"; X2
LN:   M2 = (X2 − X0)/(Y1 + Y2):PAUSE "New activity"; M2
LN:   M = (M1 + M2)/2:PRINT "Averaged"; M
L2·:  INPUT "Present ACT"; X3, "Target ACT"; X4
LN:   PAUSE "Heparin (U)",:PRINT ((X4 − X3)/M)*W*100
LN:   IF X1 < 450 GOTO L1
```

```
LN:   PRINT "Time of drawing sample at"
LN:   GOSUB ··· to time lapse program no. 2 ···
LN:   HL = ABS ((0.693*TL)/(LN (X1 − X0) − LN (X2 − X0))
LN:   PRINT "Apparent 1/2 life"; HL; "min"
L1·:  WAIT 0: PRINT "To repeat press R – else N"
LN:   R$ = INKEY$: IF R$ = "" GOTO L1
LN:   WAIT 150: IF R$ = "Y" LET X1 = 0: GOTO L2
LN:   INPUT "Heparin reversal: ACT?"; X5
LN:   PR = ((X5 − X0)/M)*W*0.6
LN:   PRINT "Protamine"; PR; "mg"
LN:   INPUT "Given at"; TS$: GOSUB ··· to time lapse program ···
L3·:  WAIT 0: PRINT "PRINT OUT? Y/N"
LN:   Z$ = INKEY$: IF Z$ = "" GOTO L3
LN:   IF Z$ = "N" GOTO L5
LN:   INPUT "Name?"; N$, "Initials"; C$, "Hosp no"; H$, "Reversed
      ACT"; X6
LN:   TEXT: CSIZE 2: COLOR 0
LN:   LPRINT "Name " + C$ + " " + N$": LPRINT "No"; H$
LN:   GOSUB ··· use the time and date program no. 4 if desired ···
LN:   LF 1: LPRINT USING " # # # # # #.#"; "Weight kg"; W:
      LPRINT "1st ACT"; X0: LPRINT "Heparin mg/kg", Y1
LN:   LPRINT "Heparin U"; Y1*W*100: IF  Y2 > 0 THEN LPRINT
      " + extra"; Y2*W*100
LN:   LPRINT "Activity"; M: LPRINT "Protamine 0.6:1", PR: LPRINT
      "Last ACT"; X6: LF3
LN:   LPRINT "Minutes heparinized", TL: LPRINT "From"; ST$; "to"
      TS$
LN:   LF 3
L5·:  END
```

11. A *variation of the vapour pressure programme* can be used for closed circuit anaesthesia using a liquid injection technique. The method is that first described by Lin and Mostert [15]. They propose that, provided wash-in of an anaesthetic mixture is rapid (10 l/min for 5–10 min), uptake of the volatile agent is constant from an early stage, possibly because of rate limiting across the alveolus. From a knowledge of the alveolar minute volume, desired inspired concentration and fraction of this concentration absorbed, the minute consumption of vapour is calculated. This is easily converted to ml liquid per h (Avogadro's hypothesis – 1 g molecular weight occupies 24 l at RTP). Data from the data lines in programme 6 are repeated here with the addition of uptake ratios for the three drugs. Using the Radford

nomogram programme [3] an alveolar minute volume at 10 breaths per minute is proposed on which to base uptake calculations. The authors use a basal flow of about 350 ml of a N_2O/O_2 mixture with 50 ml/min more oxygen than nitrous oxide and advise using an oxygen analyser in circuit (see also Lin and Mostert [16]).

The label "L/ is assigned.

```
LN:    "L":CLEAR:PAUSE "LIQUID INJECTION"
LN:    INPUT "Wt kg?"; KG
L5·:   PAUSE "CHOOSE A NUMBER"
L1·:   WAIT 5:PRINT "Halo=1 Enflur=2 Isoflur=3"
LN:    A$=INKEY$:IF INKEY$="" GOTO L1
LN:    IF A$="1" RESTORE L2
LN:    IF A$="2" RESTORE L3
LN:    IF A$="3" RESTORE L4
LN:    AA=VAL A$:IF (AA<1) OR (AA>3) THEN L5
L2·:   DATA "Halothane", 197.4, 1.86, .74 .5
L3·:   DATA "Ethrane", 184.5, 1.52, 1.68, .4
L4·:   DATA "Forane", 184.5, 1.49, 1.15, .4
LN:    READ N$, MW, SG, MC, AR
LN:    PAUSE N$; "Selected"
LN:    TV=2.7476+8.0305*KG
LN:    RR=7.5395+103.2556/KG
LN:    MV=TV*RR:AV=MV-KG*22  ···(Dead space taken as 2.2 ml/
       kg)···
LN:    WAIT:PRINT "Set T.V.(ml)"; INT (MV/10); "@ 10 bpm"
LN:    WAIT 250:PRINT "Alv Min Vol="; INT AV; "ml/min"
LN:    VV=MW/(SG*24)  ···(ml liquid giving 1 l vapour)···
LN:    MR=AV*MC*AR*10 ^ -2  ··(minute requirement of vapour at
       MAC)···
LN:    LV=MR*60*VV*10 ^ -3 ···(liquid volume per h at MAC)···
LN:    LL=LV/MC ···(liquid volume per h at 1%)···
LN:    PRINT USING " # # # . # # "; "Minute requirement"; MR
LN:    PRINT "Pure vapour @ MAC":PRINT "Liquid ml/hr MAC"; LV
LN:    PRINT "Liquid ml/hr @ 1%"; LL
LN:    PRINT N$+ "at"; MC; "%"; "needs":PRINT LV; "ml liquid per
       h"
L6·:   WAIT 0:PRINT "Reset % Y/N"
LN:    N$=INKEY$:IF N$="" GOTO L6
LN:    IF N$="N" GOTO L7
LN:    INPUT "New %?"; NC:WAIT 150
LN:    LM=LL·NC:PRINT "At"; NC; ">"; LM; "ml/h"
L7·:   END
```

12. This short program will calculate the interval in minutes between any two time entries in a 24-h period. Entries must be made using the 24-h day system, entries being 1 or more figures, i.e. 5 min past midnight can be written as 5, 05, 005 or 0005. Elapsed time periods of less than 1 h may be entered as the clock minute hand readings even if the start time is greater than the stop time, i.e. starting at 45 and stopping at 15 will give an elapsed time of 30 min.

This unit may be used to calculate the duration of an anaesthetic, the duration of action of a drug, peak response times, etc. It has not been labelled, as it will probably be accessed by a GOSUB/RETURN routine as is the calendar/time program no.4. In the version given here *starting time* is ST\$ and *stopping time* is TS\$. The *time lapse* is TL which is printed out and may be used in the programme returned to. The times from a starting point to various stages in a procedure can be calculated by re-entering the value for TS\$ and deriving a new TL value. The first two lines are *redundant* unless used as an independent program.

```
LN:    "(LABEL)":CLEAR:PAUSE "TIME LAPSE"
LN:    INPUT "START?"; ST$, "STOP?"; TS$
L1·:   IF LEN ST$ < 4 LET ST$ = "0" + ST$ : GOTO L1
L2·:   IF LEN TS$ < 4 LET TS$ = "0" + TS$ : GOTO L2
LN:    A$ = RIGHT$ (ST$,2)
LN:    B$ = LEFT$ (ST$,2)
LN:    HS = VAL B$*60
LN:    T1 = VAL A$ + HS
LN:    C$ = RIGHT$ (TS$,2)
LN:    D$ = LEFT$ (TTSS$,2)
LN:    SH = VAL D/C*60
LN:    T2 = VAL C$ + SH
LN:    TL = T2 - T1
LN:    IF TL < 0 GOSUB LS
LN:    PRINT "TIME LAPSE"; TL; "MIN"
LN:    RETURN
LS·:   IF SH = 0 AND HS = 0 LET T1 = 60 - T1 : GOTO LS1
LN:    T1 = 1440 - T1
LS1·:  TL = T2 + T1 : RETURN
```

13. Finding what is stored in computer memory is made easy by *creating a menu* that runs automatically when switched on. It starts with line 1 and the command ARUN. When using this program make sure that subsequent programs start on a line number above 20.

```
 1:  ARUN:CLS:BEEP 2, 50, 250:BEEP 1, 21, 500:WAIT 0
 2:  PRINT "LIST PROGRAMS – Y/N"
 3:  Z$=INKEY$:IF Z$="" GOTO 2
 4:  IF Z$="N" GOTO 20
 5:  WAIT 150:PRINT "A:B.S.A."
 6:  PRINT "S:SWAN GANZ"
 7:  PRINT "D:IV DRUG DRIPS"
 8:  PRINT "G:RADFORD NOMOGRAM"
 9:  PRINT "H:H – L BYPASS"
10:  PRINT "K:CLOCK"
11:  PRINT "Z:VAPOUR PRESSURES"
12:  PRINT "C:HEPARIN"
13:  PRINT "V:SET VENTILATOR"
14:  PRINT "L:LIQUID INJECTION"
20:  END
```

Q. Greek Alphabet

α	alpha	ι	iota	ρ	rho
β	beta	κ	kappa	$\Sigma\,\sigma$	sigma
γ	gamma	λ	lambda	τ	tau
$\Delta\,\delta$	delta	μ	my	υ	upsilon
ε	epsilon	ν	ny	φ	phi
ζ	zeta	ξ	xi	χ	chi
η	eta	o	omicron	ψ	psi
$\theta\,\vartheta$	theta	π	pi	ω	omega

References

1. Amiel-Tison C, Barrier G, Shnider SM, Levinson G, Hughes SC, Stefani SJ (1982) A new neurologic and adaptive capacity scoring system for evaluating obstetric medications in full-term newborns. Anesthesiology 56: 340–350

1 a. Boidin MP, Erdman WE, Faithful NS (1986) The role of ascorbic acid in etomidate toxicity. Eur J Anaesth 3: 417–422

2. Bull BS, Huse WM, Brauer FS, Korpman RA (1975) Heparin therapy during extracorporeal circulation II. J Thorac Cardiovasc Surg 69: 685–689

3. Crawford JD, Terry ME, Rourke GM (1950) Simplification of drug dosage calculation by application of the surface area principle. Pediatrics 5: 783

4. Cruchley PA, Kaplan JA, Hug CC, Nagle D (1983) Non-cardiac surgery in patients with prior myocardial revascularization. Can Anaesth Soc J 30: 629

5. Drummond JC (1985) MAC for halothane, enflurane and isoflurane in the New Zealand white rabbit: a test for the validity of MAC determinations. Anesthesiology 62: 336–338

6. Du Bois D, Du Bois EF (1916) A formula to estimate the approximate surface area if height and weight are known. Arch Intern Med 17: 863

7. Gardner RM (1981) Direct blood pressure measurement – dynamic response requirements. Anesthesiology 54: 227–236

8. Goldman L, Caldera DL, Nussbaum SR, et al (1977) Multifactorial index of cardiac risk in non-cardiac surgical procedures. N Eng J Med 297: 845

9. Gray TC (1954) Disintegration of the nervous system. Ann R Coll Surg Engl 15: 402

10. Haycock GB, Schwartz GJ, Wisotsky DH (1978) Geometric method for measuring body surface area: A height-weight formula validated in infants, children and adults. J Paed 93: 62–66

11. Kelman GR, Nunn JF (1966) Nomograms for correction of blood PO_2, PCO_2, pH and base excess for time and temperature. J Appl Physiol 21: 1484

12. Kelten JG, Perrault RA, Blajehman MA (1983) Substitution of the "Group and screen" for the full cross match in elective operations. Can Anaesth Soc J 30: 641

13. Lee HA (1976) Intravenous nutrition: Techniques and principles. S Afr Med J 50: 1725

14. Leigh JM (1985) Variation on a theme: splitting ratio. Anaesthesia 40: 70–72

15. Lin C-Y, Mostert JW (1977) Inspired O_2 and N_2O concentrations in essentially closed circuits. Anaesthetist 26: 514

16. Lin C-Y, Mostert JW, Benson DW (1980) Closed circle systems: A new direction in the practice of anesthesia. Acta Anaesth Scand 24: 354

17. Lowe HJ, Ernst EA (1981) The quantitative practice of anesthesia. Williams and Wilkins, Baltimore

18. Lunn JN (1985) Preventable anaesthetic mortality and morbidity. Anaesthesia 40: 79

19. Moffat JA, Milne B (1983) Pharmacokinetics in anaesthesia. Can Anaesth Soc J 30: 300–307
20. Mushin WW, Galloon S (1960) The concentration of anaesthetics in closed circuits with special reference to halothane. III. Clinical aspects. Br J Anaesth 32: 324
21. Olsson AK, Lindahl SGE (1985) Ventilation, dynamic compliance and ventilatory response to CO_2. Anaesthesia 40: 229–236
22. Prorok JJ, Trostle D (1984) Operative risk of general surgical procedures in patients with previous myocardial revascularization. Surg Gynaecol Obstet 159: 214
23. Prys-Roberts C, Hug CC (1984) Pharmacokinetics of anaesthesia. Blackwell, Oxford
24. Radford EP (1945) Ventilation standards for use in artificial ventilation. J Appl Physiol 7: 451–460
25. Rogers RC, Hill GE (1978) Equations for vapour pressure versus temperature: Derivation and use of the antoine equation on a hand-held programmable calculator. Br J Anaesth 50: 415–424
26. Scanlon JW, Brown WU, Weiss JB, Alper MH (1974) Neurobehavioral response of newborn infants after maternal epidural anesthesia. Anesthesiology 40: 121
27. Shappel SD, Lenfant CJM (1972) Adaptive, genetic and iatrogenic alternations of the oxyhaemoglobin-dissociation curve. Anesthesiology 37: 133
28. Steen PA, Tinker JH, Tarhan S (1978) Myocardial reinfarction after anesthesia and surgery. JAMA 239: 2566
29. Stoeckel H (1985) Quantitation, modelling and control in anaesthesia. Thieme, Stuttgart
30. Strunin L, Davies JM (1983) The liver and anaesthesia. Can Anaesth Soc J 30: 208–217
31. Sugiura K, Muraoka K, Chishiki T, Baba M (1983) The Edinburgh-2 coma scale: a new scale for assessing impaired consciousness. Neurosurgery 12: 411–415
32. Talbot HB, Sobel EH, McArthur JW, Crawford JD (1952) Functional endocrinogy from birth through adolescence. Harvard University Press, Cambridge
33. Towler CM, Garret RT, Sear JW (1982) Althesin infusions for maintenance of anaesthesia. Anaesthesia 37: 428. *See also* Anaesthesia 38 Supplement (Total intravenous anaesthesia, July 1983)
34. Van Rooyen JM, Offermeier J (1985) Pharmacokinetics of the benzodiazepines. S Afr Med J 26: Supplement
35. West JB (1970) Ventilation/blood flow and gas exchange, 2nd edn. Blackwell Scientific, Oxford